O A O L
OXFORD AMERICAN ONCOLOGY LIBRARY

Prostate Cancer

O A O L
OXFORD AMERICAN ONCOLOGY LIBRARY

Prostate Cancer

Primo N. Lara, Jr., MD

Professor of Medicine
Division of Hematology-Oncology
Department of Internal Medicine
University of California Davis School of Medicine

Associate Director for Translational Research
University of California Davis Cancer Center
Sacramento, CA

OXFORD
UNIVERSITY PRESS

OXFORD
UNIVERSITY PRESS

Oxford University Press, Inc., publishes works that further
Oxford University's objective of excellence
in research, scholarship, and education.

Oxford New York
Auckland Cape Town Dar es Salaam Hong Kong Karachi
Kuala Lumpur Madrid Melbourne Mexico City Nairobi
New Delhi Shanghai Taipei Toronto

With offices in
Argentina Austria Brazil Chile Czech Republic France Greece
Guatemala Hungary Italy Japan Poland Portugal Singapore
South Korea Switzerland Thailand Turkey Ukraine Vietnam

Copyright © 2011 by Oxford University Press, Inc.

Published by Oxford University Press, Inc.
198 Madison Avenue, New York, New York 10016
www.oup.com

Oxford is a registered trademark of Oxford University Press

Library of Congress Cataloging-in-Publication Data

Prostate cancer / Primo N. Lara Jr.
   p. ; cm. -- (Oxford American oncology library)
Includes bibliographical references and index.
ISBN 978-0-19-975478-6 (pbk. : alk. paper)
1. Prostate—Cancer. I. Lara, Primo N. II. Series: Oxford American oncology library.
[DNLM: 1. Prostatic Neoplasm—diagnosis—Handbooks. 2. Prostatic Neoplasms—
therapy—Handbooks. WJ 39]
RC280.P7P742242 2011
616.99'463—dc22   2010051004

9 8 7 6 5 4 3 2
Printed in the United States of America
on acid-free paper

Dedication

This volume is dedicated to my beautiful and supportive wife, Elizabeth ("Queennie"), and to my sons, Matthew and Joshua.

Mama Merle—this one's for you, too.

Preface

The clinical management of prostate cancer—from screening all the way to end-of-life care—has never been more complex. As the biological basis for the disease continues to be defined through carefully conducted laboratory investigations, clinical care has also evolved to become truly multidisciplinary, involving the efforts of urologic oncologists, radiologists, pathologists, molecular biologists, radiation oncologists, and medical oncologists, among many others.

All of this is occurring in an environment that is in constant flux. Emerging data from the laboratory or from observational trials are now being translated into clinical applications, with many recent studies yielding results that are simultaneously exciting and confusing. Controversy continues to hamper the field where zealots can find convincing arguments to back up their assertions from the very same dataset that opponents are able to mount counterarguments. This phenomenon has been seen in recent studies of prostate cancer screening, chemoprevention, and therapy.

It is in this context that we present this mini-textbook entitled "Prostate Cancer." I believe that this handbook arrives at a very opportune time. The simple format and style of this volume helps cut through the clutter and din of the voluminous data crowding the field. It provides a clear and concise snapshot of the complexities surrounding prostate cancer, from disease epidemiology to its relevant biology, and all the way to the myriad clinical strategies available to the practicing physician.

In order to mirror the multidisciplinary nature of prostate cancer care, I have invited many of my colleagues representing various disciplines from the UC Davis Cancer Center to assist me in developing the content for this book. The result is this handy volume—a component of the Oxford American Oncology Library—that we hope will provide the practicing clinician involved in the care of the prostate cancer patient, as well as other interested and enlightened readers, an easy-to-read, accessible, but comprehensive reference on this malignancy.

This volume would not have been possible without the expert editorial assistance of Nina Bai, Luba Goldin, and Staci Hou at Oxford University Press, outstanding copyediting by Aloysius Raj and the team at Newgen Imaging Systems, and the efforts of my administrative assistant Xong Vang at the Division of Hematology-Oncology, UC Davis School of Medicine.

In the end, we hope that this effort ultimately benefits the prostate cancer patient and his family. Truly, it is for those folks that we have dedicated our careers, and for whom the wonders of scientific discovery promise even better outcomes.

Primo N. Lara, Jr., MD
Editor

Contents

Contributors

Regina Gandour-Edwards, MD

Professor
Department of Pathology
University of California Davis School
of Medicine
Sacramento, CA

Brian Hu, MD

Department of Urology
University of California Davis School
of Medicine
Sacramento, CA

Theresa Koppie, MD

Assistant Professor
Department of Urology
University of California Davis School
of Medicine
Sacramento, CA

Hao G. Nguyen MD, PhD

Department of Urology
University of California Davis School
of Medicine
Sacramento, CA

Chong-Xian Pan, MD, PhD

Assistant Professor
Division of Hematology-Oncology
Department of Internal Medicine
University of California Davis School
of Medicine
University of California Davis Cancer
Center
Sacramento, CA

Prabhu Rajappa, MD

Division of Hematology-Oncology
Department of Internal Medicine
University of California Davis School
of Medicine
University of California Davis Cancer
Center
Sacramento, CA

Jennifer Marie Suga, MD, MPH

Division of Hematology-Oncology
Department of Internal Medicine
University of California Davis School
of Medicine
University of California Davis Cancer
Center
Sacramento, CA

Sinisa Stanic, MD

Department of Radiation Oncology
University of California Davis School
of Medicine
University of California Davis Cancer
Center
Sacramento, CA

Richard K. Valicenti, MD

Professor and Chair
Department of Radiation Oncology
University of California Davis School
of Medicine
University of California Davis Cancer
Center
Sacramento, CA

Genevieve H. Von Thesling, MD

Capt., USAF, MC, MD
Flight Surgeon/ Beale AFB
Beale, AFB, CA

Chapter 1

Prostate Cancer: Overview, Epidemiology, and Risk Factors

Primo N. Lara, Jr.

Prostate cancer is a very common malignant disease characterized by clonal proliferation of malignant cells derived from the glandular epithelium of the prostate. It is also an endocrine-mediated cancer that typically has a long natural history. Thus, many men may not necessarily require treatment, even if found to have early-stage disease. A substantial number of men do not die prematurely nor have a reduced quality of life if the cancer is left untreated. Current treatments can also result in significant morbidity.

Furthermore, the disease is characterized by a spectrum of interconnected and sometimes overlapping clinical contexts. Figure 1.1 illustrates these various clinical contexts relevant to current prostate cancer management. These considerations have led to some clinical challenges, including hotly contested debates on the value of screening and how to identify those at highest risk for cancer-related death.

Epidemiology

Prostate cancer is the most common cancer in men in the United States, with over 192,000 cases estimated in 2009. Prostate cancer accounts for 25% of all incident cases in men. It is a also leading cause of oncologic death, second only to lung cancer, resulting in approximately 27,000 deaths annually.[1]

Fortunately, prostate cancer is also a fairly indolent disease and therefore is characterized by a protracted clinical course. Between 1996 and 2004, approximately 90% of all new prostate cancer cases were clinically diagnosed at either a local or regional (i.e., nonmetastatic) stage. For those patients with early-stage disease, 5-year relative survival rates approached 100%. Following a peak in the incidence of prostate cancer in the mid-1990s—attributed to widespread use of prostate-specific antigen (PSA) testing in the broad population—there has been a marked decrease, by 4.4% per year, from 2001 to 2005.[2] This is likely due to the exhaustion of all incident cases present in the general population pool that were detectable by PSA testing.

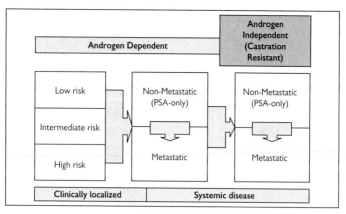

Figure 1.1 Diagrammatic Representation of the Various Clinical Contexts of Prostate Cancer

Prostate cancer is a disease of older men. According to the National Cancer Institute's Surveillance Epidemiology and Results (SEER) database, the median age at diagnosis is approximately 67 years of age.[3] The majority of patients are diagnosed at over the age of 65; in the United States, most of these patients are initially found to have organ-confined disease. The age-adjusted incidence rate, based on cases diagnosed in 2003–2007 from 17 SEER geographic areas, was 156.9 per 100,000 men per year. Prevalence of the disease in the United States as of January 1, 2007 was approximately 2,276,112 men, inclusive of patients who have had a prior diagnosis and are presumptively cured.

Risks

The lifetime risk of prostate cancer is estimated to be 1 in 6. In contrast, the risk of death due to metastatic disease is about 1 in 30, reflecting the relatively indolent nature of the disease. Approximately 80% of men who reach 80 years of age will have prostate cancer. The following risk factors have been described for this malignancy:

- **Age.** Risk steadily increases with age. In autopsy series, occult prostate cancer was seen in 29% of 30- to 40-year-old men and 64% of 60- to 70-year-old men.
- **Family history.** A positive family history increases the risk of prostate cancer. A first-degree relative who is diagnosed by age 50 increases a subject's risk sevenfold. Risk exponentially increases as more family members are affected. Screening in those individuals with a strong family history (defined as "high risk") should be considered beginning at age 40. Although there are several published reports on suspected familial genes related to prostate cancer risk, no genetic tests have been validated, and none is therefore commercially

available. In a study among 44,788 pairs of twins in Sweden, Denmark, and Finland, 42% of prostate cancers were attributed to heredity, whereas 58% were attributed to environmental causes. In the general population, it is estimated that less than 10% of all prostate cancer cases are attributable to hereditary cancer. The role of specific gene activity and molecular mechanisms remain unclear.

- **Race and geography.** Disparities occur in the distribution of prostate cancer across racial and ethnic groups. The incidence per 100,000 according to race is as follows: Asians, 82; Caucasians, 150; and African Americans, 224. Prostate cancer incidence rates are highest in Sweden, intermediate in the United States and most of Europe, and lowest in Taiwan and Japan. In the United States, prostate cancer occurs 60% more commonly in African Americans than in Caucasian Americans. Even more striking is the observation that African Americans tend to be diagnosed at a more advanced stage. Interestingly, African males living in Africa have a low incidence of prostate cancer, but the incidence increases when they immigrate to the United States. It is hypothesized that environmental factors may potentially account for this phenomenon.

- **Diet and lifestyle.** Dietary and lifestyle-related factors contribute to the risk of prostate cancer. Prospective dietary studies of tomato or lycopene (a dietary carotenoid) suggest decreased risk (approximately 20%–30% risk reduction). In a study of men fed tomato sauce–based pasta entrées three weeks prior to prostatectomy, there was a reduction in the serum PSA level, and increased lycopene levels were detected in the blood and the prostate, associated with decreased oxidative genomic damage in leukocytes and prostate cells. In the Health Professionals Follow-up Study of 51,529 subjects, increased total fat, animal fat, and red meat intake were associated with a higher risk of prostate cancer. Similarly, in the Physicians' Health Study, high red meat intake correlated with increased prostate cancer risk. It is believed that red meats cooked at high temperatures or broiled on charcoal grills can cause heterocyclic aromatic amine and polycyclic aromatic hydrocarbon carcinogen formation. It is known that the heterocyclic amine carcinogen, 2-amino-1-methyl-6-phenylimidazo[4,5-b]pyridine (PhIP), causes prostate cancer when fed to rats.

- **Androgens.** Androgens are known to facilitate the development and progression of prostate cancer. Prostate cancer initially responds to androgen deprivation therapy (i.e., castration). Indirect evidence for androgens contributing to prostate cancer risk can be culled from studies in prepubertal castrates. Clinical evaluation of Ottoman court eunuchs revealed that the subjects' prostates were markedly atrophied (prepubertal in size). In a study of Chinese eunuchs, the prostate was completely impalpable in 21 of 26 subjects, and very small in the other five. None of these eunuchs ever developed prostate cancer. However, the precise levels of androgen—either intracellularly or systemically—that correspond to a particular risk of developing prostate cancer have not been defined.

Prevention of Prostate Cancer

The concept of prostate cancer prevention hinges on the ability of a therapeutic agent to reverse, suppress, or prevent the prostatic carcinogenic process, thus blocking the development of clinically manifest disease. This agent should ideally be of low toxicity, high efficacy, and targeted toward a group of individuals that have "sufficiently increased risk for developing prostate cancer for which chemoprevention is appropriate and cost-effective".[4] The protracted natural history of prostate cancer makes it an ideal tumor against which chemoprevention strategies can be deployed. Furthermore, the multistep pathogenesis and long evolution from premalignant to malignant makes the idea of prevention achievable.

In the Selenium and Vitamin E Cancer Prevention Trial (SELECT), 35,000 men were randomized to selenium, vitamin E, selenium and vitamin E, or placebo in a double-blind fashion.[5] These antioxidants had been shown in preclinical and epidemiologic data to have an impact on prostate cancer risk, as well as overall cancer mortality. Begun in 2001, the study was closed early by its data safety monitoring committee in September 2008 on the grounds that no benefit had been seen nor was likely to occur from taking vitamin E and selenium. At a median follow-up of 5.46 years, there was no difference in the incidence of prostate cancer in any of the groups. There was a nonsignificant increase in prostate cancer diagnoses in the vitamin E arm, and a nonsignificant increase in type II diabetes was seen in the selenium arm. The lack of benefit from vitamin E was also confirmed in the Physicians Health Study II, which showed no difference in the risk of prostate or any other cancer in men randomized to daily vitamin E supplementation.[6] In patients with a history of high-grade prostatic intraepithelial neoplasia (PIN), a large trial from the Southwest Oncology Group also showed no benefit for selenium supplementation in preventing the development of invasive prostate cancer.

Two large, randomized, controlled trials have shown benefit from 5-α reductase inhibitors in the prevention of prostate cancer. The Prostate Cancer Prevention Trial (PCPT) evaluated 18,882 men over the age of 55 and assigned them to finasteride 5 mg daily or placebo. This was a true primary prevention trial, as all the men in the study group had normal digital rectal exams (DREs), PSA levels of less than 3.0 ng/mL, and no benign prostatic hypertrophy (BPH) symptoms. Biopsies were recommended if the PSA (adjusted for effects of finasteride) reached 4 ng/mL or for an abnormal DRE. Biopsies were performed in all men at the end of the study. The results showed a 25% relative risk reduction in the prevalence of prostate cancer in the treatment group after the 7-year treatment period.[7,8] Although at the time of initial data analysis there was concern that the use of finasteride increased the development of prostate cancers with Gleason's score of 7 or higher, a reanalysis of the data in late 2007, which accounted for changes in prostate volume, did not confirm this concern.[9] Analyses of the same data by two other groups show that finasteride use does not increase the rate of high-grade prostate cancer.[10,11] The most common side effects noted in the trial included a decrease in ejaculate, erectile dysfunction, loss of libido, and gynecomastia. As one might expect, symptoms of BPH—urinary frequency, urgency, and retention—were fewer in the treatment group.

The Reduction by Dutasteride of Prostate Cancer Events Trial (REDUCE) trial included 8,121 men at high risk for the development of prostate cancer by virtue of PSA levels of 2.5 or 3 (depending on age) to 10 ng/mL. It was an international, randomized, controlled trial in which men who had undergone a negative prostate biopsy within 6 months of enrollment were randomized to dutasteride or placebo for a period of 4 years. Patients received biopsies after 2 and 4 years of follow-up. Results were similar to that of the PCPT, with a 23% relative risk reduction in the number of prostate cancer cases in the treatment group and no significant increase in the number of high-grade lesions. Because all patients had a biopsy prior to enrollment, the chance of diagnosing a preexisting cancer was significantly decreased when compared with the PCPT. The most common side effects seen were erectile dysfunction, decreased libido, and gynecomastia.[12]

Thus, both the PCPT and REDUCE trials showed that 5-α reductase inhibitor therapy can reduce the risk of a prostate cancer diagnosis by approximately 22%–25%. A number of clinicians are now comfortable recommending 5-α reductase inhibitor therapy in select individuals. These include men at high risk for prostate cancer (e.g., positive family history or high PSA but negative biopsy), men with lower urinary tract symptoms from BPH who require symptomatic therapy, and highly motivated men who are extremely concerned with their personal risk of developing prostate cancer. Regardless, the wide clinical application of these findings remains controversial. The role of selective estrogen receptor modulators, nonsteroidal anti-inflammatory drugs, vitamin D, lycopene, and others in preventing prostate cancer are currently being investigated.[13]

Prostate-specific Antigen

Prostate-specific antigen (PSA) is 34 kD glycoprotein produced almost exclusively by prostate epithelium. The PSA gene is located at chromosome 19q13. The normal physiologic role of PSA is to liquefy seminal fluid coagulum, allowing for the proper environment for sperm motility and survival. Although PSA levels are highest in seminal fluid, a small amount "backwashes" into the general circulation and is detectable by commercially available assays. It is the PSA level in serum that is clinically employed to screen for and monitor prostate cancer activity.

Under normal conditions, a proenzyme (proPSA) is produced and processed to generate active PSA. Active PSA is further degraded to the inactive PSA, which enters the bloodstream as unbound PSA (free PSA). A small amount of active PSA diffuses into the circulation and forms complexes with two protease inhibitors, α1-antichymotrypsin and α2-macroglobulin. Prostate cancer lacks the normal prostate gland structure, with disruption of the basal membrane.

Therefore, a larger fraction of proPSA, active PSA, and several truncated PSA forms escapes proteolysis, diffuses into circulation, and forms complexes with protease inhibitors (bound PSA). Thus, the percentage of free PSA is lower in patients with prostate cancer. The ratio of free PSA has been used to facilitate risk stratification in prostate cancer screening.

Prostate-specific antigen levels are higher in patients with larger prostate glands, such as those with BPH or prostatic inflammation (e.g., viral or bacterial prostatitis). Prostatic massage, DRE, and sexual activity can also slightly increase the PSA level, but not in a clinically significant manner. Importantly, the PSA test should not be considered a diagnostic test for prostate cancer; instead, it is just another clinical tool used to identify men who have a reasonable chance of harboring cancer and for whom a biopsy is being contemplated.

The absolute level of PSA, although reflective of normal and/or malignant prostate volume or activity, is actually less useful than the rate of PSA rise. This rate of rise is often clinically translated into *PSA velocity* or *PSA doubling time*, with many studies showing that a steeper PSA slope is associated with worse clinical outcomes, such as increased recurrence risk following curative therapy.[14] PSA doubling time is defined as the time it takes for a PSA value to double based on an exponential growth pattern while PSA velocity is simply the rate of PSA change over time. PSA doubling time is traditionally calculated using the "log-slope method", wherein the natural log (ln) of each PSA measurement is plotted versus time on a Cartesian coordinate system plot (x-y axis), and then measuring the slope of the linear regression (m) through the data points. The doubling time is subsequently calculated by dividing ln 2 by m, the slope of the linear regression. Since this method is relatively cumbersome, clinicians typically use one of many PSA doubling time calculators available on the internet instead.

In the past, an absolute PSA level of 4 ng/mL or lower was considered within the "normal range." However, up to 15%–20 % of men with PSA at or below 4.0 ng/mL can harbor prostate cancer, some of which are high-grade and therefore, high risk. Conversely, in men with PSA levels between 4 and 10 ng/mL, only 25%–35% are expected to have prostate cancer at biopsy. Thus, there is no single cutoff PSA level that can simultaneously yield high diagnostic sensitivity (correctly identify patients who do have cancer) and specificity (correctly identify patients who do not have cancer).

The fact that PSA levels also tend to increase with age has led to the development of age-adjusted PSA tables, but these are of modest clinical utility. Other attempts to improve the PSA test include using PSA density, which accounts for the relationship between PSA and prostate volume); using free PSA level (higher percent free levels are associated with benign prostate conditions); and lowering the PSA cutoff level to increase the cancer detection rate (at the expense of overdiagnosis and false-positive results). Thus, absolute PSA levels—which linearly correlate with a greater likelihood of a prostate cancer diagnosis—are of limited value in the diagnostic setting.

The widespread use of the PSA test has visibly changed the prostate cancer landscape over the past 25 years. Prior to the 1980s, most prostate cancers were diagnosed at a locally advanced or metastatic stage. Since the PSA era, less than 5% of all new prostate cancers are diagnosed at a metastatic stage. In fact, approximately 70%–80% of men with prostate cancer are now found to have clinically nonpalpable (or T1c) disease—presumably more curable—detected largely by an abnormal or rising PSA test. Despite this change, the role of PSA in screening for prostate cancer remains highly controversial; this issue is discussed elsewhere in this book.

In patients who already have a diagnosis of prostate cancer, the PSA test is useful in monitoring disease activity and subsequently, in therapeutic decision-making. For example, a detectable PSA in a man who has undergone a radical prostatectomy almost certainly will indicate persistent disease. Some of these patients may be offered other "salvage" therapies such as radiation therapy, ostensibly to cure the disease.

Treatment decisions are not typically made on the basis of a single follow-up PSA test. It is in this context that several other clinical factors, including the PSA doubling time, patient comorbidities and desires, and other findings (e.g., from imaging studies), are used to develop a therapeutic plan. In the National Comprehensive Cancer Network (NCCN) Clinical Practice Guidelines,[15] sub-groups of men with rising PSA can be considered for therapeutic changes in the following clinical contexts:

- **For men currently on watchful waiting.** A PSA level that has doubled in less than 3 years or a PSA velocity (change in PSA level over time) of more than 0.75 ng/mL per year, or a prostate biopsy showing evidence of worsening cancer.

- **For men status post radical prostatectomy.** A PSA level that does not fall below the limits of detection after surgery or is at a detectable level (>0.3 ng/mL) that increases on two or more subsequent measurements after having no detectable PSA.

- **For men who have had other initial therapy, such as radiation therapy with or without hormonal therapy.** A PSA level that has risen by 2 ng/mL or more after having no detectable PSA or a very low PSA level.

References

1. Jemal A, Siegel R, Ward E, et al. Cancer Statistics 2009. *CA Cancer J Clin* *2009*;59:225–249.

2. Smith DS, Humphrey PA, Catalona WJ. The early detection of prostate carcinoma with prostate specific antigen: The Washington University experience. *Cancer 1997*;80(9):1853–1856.

3. Altekruse SF, Kosary CL, Krapcho M, et al., eds. *SEER Cancer Statistics Review, 1975–2007*. Bethesda, MD: National Cancer Institute, 2009. Available online at http://seer.cancer.gov/csr/1975_2007/, based on November 2009 SEER data submission, posted to the SEER web site, 2010.

4. Klein E. Screening and prevention of prostate cancer in the post-randomized trial era. *Genitourin Cancers Symp Proc* 2010:10–12.

5. Lippman S, Klein EA, Goodman PJ, et al. Effect of selenium and vitamin E on risk of prostate cancer and other cancers: The Selenium and Vitamin E Cancer Prevention Trial (SELECT). *JAMA* 2009;301(1):39–51.

6. Gaziano JM, Glynn RJ, Christen WG, et al. Vitamins E and C in the prevention of prostate and total cancer in men: The Physicians' Health Study II randomized controlled trial. *JAMA* 2009;301(1): 52–62.

7. Thompson IM, Goodman PJ, Tangen CM, et al. The influence of finasteride on the development of prostate cancer. *N Engl J Med* 2003;349:215–224.

8. Thompson IM, Pauler DK, Goodman PJ, et al. Prevalence of prostate cancer among men with a prostate-specific antigen level ≤ 4.0 ng per milliliter. *N Engl J Med 2004*;350(22):2239–2246.

9. Lucia MS, Epstein JI, Goodman PJ, et al. Finasteride and high-grade prostate cancer in the Prostate Cancer Prevention Trial. *J Natl Cancer Inst* 2007; 99(18):1375–1383.

10. Redman MW, Tangen CM, Goodman PJ, et al. Finasteride does not increase the risk of high-grade prostate cancer: A bias-adjusted modeling approach. *Cancer Prev Res (Phila Pa)* 2009;1(3):174–181.

11. Pinsky P, Parnes H, Lucia MS, et al. Estimating rates of true high-grade disease in the Prostate Cancer Prevention Trial. *Cancer Prev Res (Phila Pa)* 2008;1(3):182–186.

12. Andriole GL, Bostwick DG, Brawley OW, et al. Effect of dutasteride on the risk of prostate cancer. *N Engl J Med* 2010;362:1192–1202.

13. Brawley OW, Lucia S, Andriole G. Chemoprevention of prostate cancer. *ASCO Education Book* 2009:62–64.

14. Carter HB, Ferrucci L, Kettermann A, et al. Detection of life-threatening prostate cancer with prostate-specific antigen velocity during a window of curability. *J Natl Cancer Inst* 2006;98(21):1521–1527.

15. National Comprehensive Cancer Network. *NCCN Clinical Practice Guidelines in Oncology™: Prostate Cancer v.2.2009*. Retrieved March 18, 2009, from http://www.nccn.org/professionals/physician_gls/PDF/prostate.pdf.

Chapter 2

Prostate Cancer Biology

Chong-Xian Pan

Initiation of the Malignant Process

As highlighted in the previous chapter, prostate cancer risk factors include advancing age as well as ethnic, genetic, hormonal, environmental, social, and dietary factors. Additionally, hereditary factors also influence risk and are likely involved in the initiation of prostatic carcinogenesis. Cohort analysis of cancer between twins showed that about 42% of prostate cancers were attributed to inheritance.[1] The risk of prostate cancer also increases as the number of first-degree relatives with prostate cancer increases. Linkage analysis and cytogenetic studies have already identified several chromosomal loci and genes that are frequently associated with prostate cancer. The gene that appears to be associated with the highest risk for hereditary prostate is *BRCA2*, a gene involved in repair of DNA. However, *BRCA2* mutations are rare in prostate cancer. Other chromosome loci mutations compellingly associated with prostate cancer include loss of chromosome 8p, 5q, 6q, 13 q, and 18, and gain of 1q, 3q, 8q24, and Xq12. Some of these chromosome loci are not associated with any specific genes, thus suggesting that noncoding transcripts, such as microRNA, may be associated with the development of prostate cancer.

Some genes, such as *CTBP2, EHBP1, KLK2* and *KLK3, LMTK2, MSMB,* and *SLC22A3* have been reported to be associated with prostate cancer. Recently, it was found that TMPRSS2-ETS family translocations, leading to overexpression of ERG and, less commonly, other members of ETS family, may be the most common cancer gene rearrangement in prostate cancer. Over the past few years, genome-wide association studies have identified many more genetic alterations—including single nucleotide polymorphisms (SNPs)—associated with prostate cancer. However, each of these loci, genes, or SNPs is associated with only a modest increase in the risk of prostate cancer. Importantly, other studies have failed to reproduce the same linkages.

Besides the above-mentioned genomic sequence changes, epigenetic changes related to prostate cancer have been well documented in over 50 genes. Differential DNA hypermethylation of adenomatous polyposis coli (*APC*), glutathione S-transferase pl (*GSTP1*), and multidrug resistance 1 (*MDR1*), *RARB2, RASSF1A* have been detected preferentially in prostate cancer as compared with noncancerous prostate tissue. Some of these epigenetic DNA methylation events apparently occur early in the development of prostate cancer. In later stages, particularly at the metastatic step, global hypomethylation with decreased methylation at specific genes such as *LINE-1* has been reported. Besides changes in DNA methylation, another epigenetic event associated with prostate carcinogenesis has been modification of histones (e.g., variances in histone acetylation). Alterations of DNA methylation and histone acetylation lead to a change in chromatin structure and, subsequently, to the expression of oncogenes and tumor-suppressor genes.

Recently, small noncoding microRNAs (miRNAs) have been found to be involved in the regulation of genes and oncogenesis. The evolutionarily conserved miRNAs bind to complementary sites within the 3' untranslated region of target mRNA and regulate gene expression via inducing degradation or translational repression. miRNA behaves like transcription factors in that one miRNA can interact with many mRNAs and affect the expression of many genes, whereas a single mRNA can be targeted by different miRNAs. It is estimated that up to a third of the protein-coding genes are potential targets for miRNA regulation.

Several approaches have been used to analyze miRNA expression, such as oligonucleotide microarray, quantitative real-time polymerase chain reaction (qRT-PCR), bead-based method, cloning miRNA serial analysis of gene expression (MiRAGE), and Northern blot assays. Several miRNAs are consistently down- or upregulated in prostate cancer cells compared with normal or benign prostate tissue. The expression profile of miRNAs can potentially distinguish prostate cancer from normal/benign prostate tissue.[2] These miRNAs contribute to prostate carcinogenesis either directly or indirectly. These miRNAs can directly (negatively) regulate proapoptotic genes or genes suppressing cell-cycle progression, cell migration, and invasion. These can also indirectly affect upregulation of oncogenic genes. Since one miRNA can regulate a group of genes and several regulatory pathways, it is fascinating to imagine a drug development strategy that yields therapeutic agents directed against miRNA for cancer therapy.

In conclusion, it takes many steps and requires multiple transformational events for normal prostate glandular epithelial cells to develop into clinically aggressive prostate cancer. This process involves genetic and epigenetic alterations that lead to loss of tumor-suppressor and housekeeping genes, activation of oncogenes, and upregulation of growth stimulatory signaling pathways. For example, loss of tumor-suppressor gene phosphate and tensin homolog-10 and GSTP1, overexpression of anti-apoptotic Bcl2, and activation of telomerase have all been documented in prostate cancer.

Prostate Cancer Stem Cells

It has been recently proposed that, like embryogenesis, most cancers originate from a small population of cells named *cancer stem cells* (CSC) or *tumor-initiating cells*. The CSC can self-renew to maintain the stem cell pool while also being capable of proliferating and differentiating into more heterogeneous cancer cells. Cancer stem cells account for a small population of cancer cells. They have been identified in both solid and hematological malignancies, suggesting their occurrence to be a common phenomenon among malignancies. In prostate cancer, the cell surface markers of prostate CSC resemble those of the basal cells of prostate gland, such as $CD133^+$, $CD44^+$, and $\alpha_2\beta_1^{hi}$. The CSC also express high levels of stemness genes, such as *OCT3/4*, *Nanog*, *Sox2*, and *BMI1*. Nevertheless, microarray analysis showed that the gene expression profile of prostate CSC is different from that of normal prostate stem cells and more differentiated cancer cells. The prostate CSC are negative for androgen receptor (AR), whereas the vast majority of more differentiated prostate cancer cells express AR. During culture or *in vivo* xenograft formation, the AR-negative CSC can differentiate into AR-positive, more differentiated cancer cells. In those cases in which the recurrent TMPRSS2-ERG fusion gene is identified in prostate cancer cells, this fusion gene could also be detected in the $CD133^+$/ $\alpha_2\beta_1^{hi}$ presumed CSC from prostate tumors, suggesting that this translocation occurs at the early stage of prostate oncogenesis and that the cell origin of prostate cancer is a stem cell.

Identification of CSC in prostate cancer may have significant impacts on management. Hormonal therapy is highly effective in the treatment of prostate cancer. However, prostate CSC do not express AR and are resistant to hormonal therapy. Even though hormonal therapy kills the sensitive, more differentiated prostate cancer cells, the resistant AR-negative CSC will proliferate and generate more cancer cells. Like any other cancer cells, prostate CSC are also chemoresistant, in that they usually remain at the quiescent state and overexpress multidrug resistant genes, such as ABC transporters. Furthermore, genetic instability allows them more easily to develop chemoresistance and evade immunotherapy.

Identification of CSC will have profound effects on the evaluation of the treatment of prostate cancer. To cure prostate cancer, prostate CSC must be eradicated. Unfortunately, so far, there is no specific and effective therapy targeting prostate CSC. Prostate CSC account for less than 1% of all prostate cancer cells. Even if all of the CSC are eradicated, the traditional approach of evaluating the response by doing imaging studies may not reflect the efficacy of therapy. Furthermore, the production of prostate-specific antigen (PSA) is highly regulated by androgen, and prostate CSC are AR-negative. Therefore, CSC may produce no or little PSA, and the commonly used approach to monitor PSA change may not work in this case.

Relevant Signaling Pathways

Abnormal signaling not only plays important roles in the development of prostate cancer, but also contributes to disease progression and development of resistance to hormonal therapy and chemotherapy. To make the analysis more complicated, many of the signaling pathways intercalate each other, and redundant pathways exist. Here, we discuss a few important pathways.

The Androgen Receptor Pathway

The androgen receptor (AR) belongs to a large family of DNA-binding transcription factors that are activated by the binding of the androgenic hormones testosterone or dihydrotestosterone. There are several domains in AR: the N-terminal regulatory domain, the middle DNA-binding domain (DBD), the C-terminal ligand binding domain (LBD), and the hinge domain located between DBD and LBD. The DBD is responsible for the binding of AR to androgen-responsive element (ARE) with the sequences of 5′-AGAACANNNTGTTCT-3′ on the promoter of androgen-responsive genes. In the absence of ligand binding, AR aggregates with chaperone proteins, such as heat-shock proteins, and remains an inactive conformation in the cytoplasm. Upon ligand binding, a conformational change leads to a dissociation from the chaperone protein and homodimerization of AR, which is followed by nuclear translocation and binding to AREs in the promoter of androgen-responsive genes to regulate gene expression. Recent studies also showed the nontranscriptional activities of AR signaling pathways.

The androgen receptor plays a central role in the initiation and propagation of prostate cancer. Even in prostate cancer that no longer responds to hormonal therapy, the role of AR is still critical in the vast majority of cells. However, despite the convincing clinical and laboratory evidence of AR in prostate cancer, activation of the AR pathway alone is insufficient in causing prostate cancer. Some other genetic or epigenetic alterations are required for the full transformation of normal prostatic epithelial cells into cancer cells. Deletion or silencing of tumor-suppressor genes and activation of oncogenes have been identified in prostate cancer cells. Like any other cancer, "the hallmarks of cancer," as reviewed by Hanahan and Weinberg, have to be fulfilled in prostate cancer.[3] Most of these "hallmarks" are not regulated by androgen(s).

PI3K/AKT Pathway

The phosphoinositide 3-kinase (PI3K)/AKT pathway plays a crucial role in transducing extracellular signals into cells. It funnels various signals from receptor-associated and non–receptor-associated tyrosine kinases (Fig. 2.1). Upon activation, the downstream serine-threonine kinase Akt phosphorylates and regulates many other proteins, kinases, transcription factors, and other regulatory factors. It is negatively regulated by the tumor-suppressor gene *PTEN*. To make things more complicated, the PI3K/AKT pathway integrates with many other signaling pathways, including the AR pathway. Phosphoinositide 3-kinases have been linked to an extraordinarily diverse group of cellular functions, including cell growth, proliferation, differentiation, motility, survival, and intracellular trafficking.

In prostate cancer, this pathway is not only involved in the initiation of prostate oncogenesis, but is also important for disease progression from localized cancer to metastasis and the development of hormone-refractory prostate cancer. For example, loss of PTEN, either through deletion, or gene silencing via epigenetic changes, or mutation, is found in up to two-thirds of prostate cancer specimens, and is associated with clinically advanced disease and poorer prognosis. Activation of the PI3K/AKT pathway is associated with development

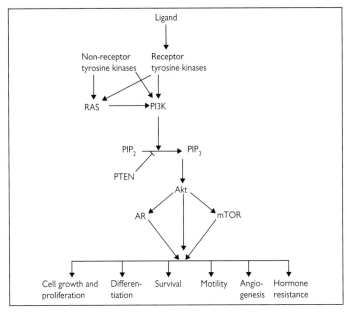

Figure 2.1 The PI3K/PTEN/AKT pathway.

of hormone-refractory and chemoresistant prostate cancer. However, as single agents, small molecules inhibiting the PI3K/AKT pathway have limited clinical activities. One possible explanation is that redundant pathways rescue the prostate cancer cells from inhibition of the PI3K/AKT pathway.

The ErbB Receptor Family

There are four members in the ErbB family receptor tyrosine kinase (RTK): epidermal growth factor receptor (EGFR or ErbB1), HER2/Neu (ErbB2), HER3 (ErbB3), and HER4 (ErbB4). Each one has an extracellular ligand-binding domain, a transmembrane domain, and an intracellular tyrosine kinase domain. Signaling of the ErbB RTK requires homo- or heterodimerization of the ErbB family members. The downstream signaling pathways include the PI3K/AKT pathway and Ras/MAPK pathway. The ErbB signaling pathway may also affect the interleukin-6 pathway, which is also shown to be involved in the development of hormone-refractory prostate cancer. Overexpression of the ErbB members, especially EGFR, is associated with poor prognosis and hormone-refractoriness of prostate cancer.

Other Pathways

Src tyrosine kinases are a group of nonreceptor tyrosine kinases. They all have in common six distinct domains, including the N-terminal Src homology domain (SH4), a unique domain, SH3, SH2, SH1 kinase domain, and the

C-terminal regulatory region. They play significant roles in transducing diverse extracellular stimuli and in crosstalk between many signaling pathways. The target genes of the Src kinases are not only involved in the transition of cell cycle from G0/G1 to S phase, but are also important in many other cellular functions such as differentiation, adhesion, and oncogenesis. In prostate cancer, Src kinases are highly expressed in the majority of specimens. They are also involved in the development of hormone-independent prostate cancer and bone metastasis.

Many other signaling pathways play important roles in prostate cancer development and disease progression. Integrins are cell surface heterodimer receptors. Each integrin receptor is composed of non–covalently bound α and β subunits. They are involved in the cell adhesion, migration, and signal transduction important for cell proliferation and apoptosis. Other growth factors, such as fibroblast growth factor, insulin-like growth factor, growth factors involved in angiogenesis, interleukin-6 (IL-6) and IL-8 were found to be involved in the development of prostate cancer and hormone-independent cancer.

Regulation of Androgen Production and Targeting for Hormonal Therapy

Since androgens play critical roles both in normal prostate development and in prostate cancer development, analysis of the regulation of androgen production will help in understanding the targets of hormonal therapy. The production of androgen is tightly regulated by the hypothalamus-pituitary-gonadal/adrenal (HPG/HPA) axis. Figure 2.2 shows the regulation of androgen production and the targets for hormonal therapy. Among the possible first-line hormonal therapies, estrogen is rarely used nowadays due to its potential complications, mainly thrombosis and pulmonary embolism. The other three options probably have similar efficacy. Luteinizing-hormone releasing-hormone (LHRH) is secreted in a pulsatile pattern. The LHRH agonists may cause the initial stimulation of LH by the pituitary, a surge of testosterone production, and a flare of symptoms. Therefore, an AR modulator is sometimes combined with an LHRH agonist during the first weeks of treatment to prevent flares. With continuous stimulation, the production of LH and, therefore, testosterone is suppressed.

Androgen receptor modulators (flutamide, bicalutamide, and nilutamide) are commonly used as second-line hormonal therapy when patients have disease progression after first-line hormonal therapy. Even though all three modulators are supposed to act at the testosterone binding site, there are slight differences among the three medications. Response sometimes can be observed when prostate cancer is treated with another AR modulator after disease progression occurs with one modulator. The use of complete androgen blockade with the combination of the first-line therapy and AR modulator is still controversial.

Although the majority of androgen is produced at the testicles, a small amount of testosterone is produced at the adrenal glands, and this can be suppressed by ketoconazole. Ketoconazole itself may have direct effects on the cancer cells. Abiraterone inhibits 17α-hydroxylase/17,20-lyase, an enzyme

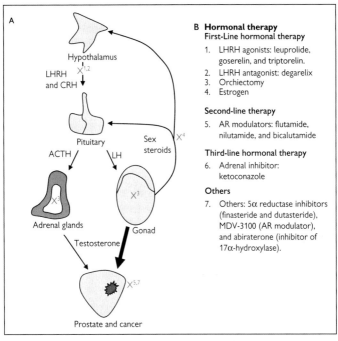

Within the figure:

A

Hypothalamus

LHRH $\times^{1,2}$
and CRH

Pituitary

ACTH

LH

Sex steroids $\times^4$

Adrenal glands $\times^3$

Gonad $\times^3$

Testosterone

Prostate and cancer $\times^{5,7}$

B **Hormonal therapy**
First-Line hormonal therapy

1. LHRH agonists: leuprolide, goserelin, and triptorelin.
2. LHRH antagonist: degarelix
3. Orchiectomy
4. Estrogen

Second-line therapy

5. AR modulators: flutamide, nilutamide, and bicalutamide

Third-line hormonal therapy

6. Adrenal inhibitor: ketoconazole

Others

7. Others: 5α reductase inhibitors (finasteride and dutasteride), MDV-3100 (AR modulator), and abiraterone (inhibitor of 17α-hydroxylase).

Figure 2.2 The hypothalamus-pituitary-gonadal/adrenal (HPG/HPA) axis and the targets for hormonal therapy in prostate cancer. **A. The regulation of testosterone production by the HPG/HPA axis.** Hypothalamus secretes **Luteinizing-hormone-releasing hormone (LHRH)** and corticotrophin releasing hormone (CRH) to stimulate pituitary that subsequently produces LH and adrenocortical tropic hormone (ACTH). LHRH is secreted in a pulsatile pattern. Upon LH stimulation, testicles produce the vast majority of testosterone where a small amount of testosterone is produced at the adrenal gland and other tissues. **B. Hormonal therapy for prostate cancer.** LHRH agonists may cause initial stimulation of pituitary to produce LH and a surge of testosterone production that may cause flare. After a few weeks, continuous stimulation of pituitary by LHRH agonist will suppress the production of LH and achieve the therapeutic purposes.

required in the cascade of androgen production from cholesterol. MDV-3100 is another AR modulator under development that works in some hormone-independent prostate cancer.

Mechanisms of Castration Resistance

Even though initially highly effective, most prostate cancer will eventually develop resistance to androgen deprivation or "hormonal" therapy. Five major mechanisms have been identified that explain such resistance:

• Overexpression or mutation of AR, or in situ synthesis of androgen by cancer cells or stromal cells, leading to extreme sensitivity to low levels of androgen or even cells that are constitutively active in the absence of androgen.

- Mutations and other alterations of AR that allow other nonandrogen steroid hormones and even AR modulators like bicalutamide to bind to and activate the AR pathway. Bicalutamide is an antiandrogen that is commonly used as a second-line hormonal therapy after disease progression with LHRH agonist. An antiandrogen withdrawal response (characterized by a decrease of PSA after withdrawal of bicalutamide), which occurs in approximately 15% of patients, suggests that bicalutamide can uncommonly activate the AR pathway.

- Other nonsteroid signaling pathways, such as insulin growth factor (IGF), HER-2/neu, and IL-6 pathways, activate the AR pathway.

- Alteration of coactivators or corepressors leads to direct activation of the AR pathway.

- Some prostate cancer cells become completely independent of the AR pathway by utilizing other pathways to stimulate prostate cancer cell growth. This is especially true in those with low or absent PSA and highly aggressive prostate cancer, as in some prostate cancer cell lines that are absent of AR expression.

Prostate cancer cells may utilize a combination of these mechanisms or redundant pathways to achieve hormone-independence or "castration-resistance". This may also explain why inhibition of single pathways (such as IL-6, mTOR, or IGF) is rarely efficacious in the clinical setting, whereas combined inhibition of multiple pathways may achieve synergistic effects.

References

1. Lichtenstein P, Holm NV, Verkasalo PK, et al. Environmental and heritable factors in the causation of cancer—analyses of cohorts of twins from Sweden, Denmark, and Finland. *N Engl J Med* 2000;343:78–85.

2. Gandellini P, Folini M, Zaffaroni N. Towards the definition of prostate cancer-related microRNAs: Where are we now? *Trends Mol Med* 2009;15:381–390.

3. Hanahan D, Weinberg RA. The hallmarks of cancer. *Cell* 2000;100:57–70.

Chapter 3

Prostate Cancer Screening

Prabhu Rajappa and Primo N. Lara, Jr.

Rationale for Prostate Cancer Screening

As noted in Chapter 1, prostate cancer is the most common malignancy in men, with one out of six men in the United States ultimately receiving this diagnosis. It is also highly prevalent, with over 2 million men in the United States currently living with the disease.[1] The majority of these cases are asymptomatic; hence, screening has been advocated by some to detect prostate cancer at a stage at which it can be cured. However, the long natural history of the disease, other competing causes of death, and the morbidities of diagnostic and therapeutic procedures for those not destined to die of prostate cancer has made broad-based screening a highly controversial issue.

The current tools used for prostate cancer screening are the digital rectal exam (DRE) and blood testing for prostate-specific antigen (PSA). There is little debate that screening via PSA and DRE results in the detection of more prostate cancers, despite the very low positive predictive value of either or both tests. Nevertheless, the effect of this early detection on prostate cancer mortality has often been called into question. Even if some lives are saved by screening, many wonder if the risks of screening outweigh the benefits to the population as a whole. Estimates of the rate of overdiagnosis (i.e., cases that never would have become clinically evident without screening) are as high as 42% .[2] Subsequent overtreatment leads to considerable anxiety and morbidity in many patients.

The economic costs of screening are also significant, including not only the cost of testing but also subsequent biopsies and other follow-up tests. Much of the controversy has been fueled by conflicting results seen in studies, which predominantly have consisted of case-control studies, epidemiologic studies, and subsequent meta-analyses. In 2009, the results of two highly anticipated large, randomized prospective trials were published. The results of these trials and their contribution to the continuing debate are described below.

Screening Tools

Digital Rectal Exam

The DRE is the oldest and most readily available technique for prostate cancer screening. The examiner feels for asymmetry or hard, nodular areas on the prostate. A positive DRE typically leads to the recommendation of a prostate biopsy. There are widely variable reported rates of sensitivity and specificity that range from 33% to 69% and 45% to 97%, respectively. Thus, a normal DRE will miss many cancers, and roughly two out of every three biopsies done for an abnormal DRE will be benign.[3] The role of DRE in prostate cancer screening is largely as a complement to PSA testing. Despite its limitations, few argue against DRE because it is of low cost and has no complications.

Prostate-specific Antigen

The development of the commercial PSA test led to its approval by the U.S. Food and Drug Administration in 1986. Since that time, screening for prostate cancer with routine PSA testing has become widespread in the United States and parts of Western Europe, despite definitive evidence (or absence) of its efficacy as a screening tool. In 2005, it was reported that 33.5% of all U.S. men aged 50–64 had undergone PSA testing in the previous year.[4] Estimates of men over 50 who have ever had PSA screening are as high as 75% .[5]

Elevated PSA levels are not specific to prostate cancer, as false positives can be seen with prostatic infection or irritation, trauma, benign prostatic hyperplasia (BPH), and recent ejaculation. The traditional cutoff for a "normal" PSA is 4 ng/mL. However, studies have demonstrated that there is a significant incidence of prostate cancer in men even with PSA levels of less than 4 ng/mL. In one study of 2,950 men who have never had an abnormal PSA or DRE, 15% had occult prostate cancer. In these men, the test had only a 20% sensitivity and 94% specificity at a cutoff of 4.1 ng/mL. As one might expect, lower thresholds of PSA increase sensitivity at the expense of specificity. A significant number of studies, as well as practitioners, use the lower threshold of 2.5–3 ng/mL, which doubles the sensitivity but lowers the specificity to less than 75% .[5]

Another significant shortcoming of the PSA test is its inability to differentiate aggressive cancers with metastatic potential from those indolent cases that probably would never have become clinically evident without screening. Numerous trials and anecdotal cases have shown that, even when PSA values are within the normal range, aggressive prostate cancer can be present. On the other hand, many men with PSA values over 4 ng/mL can go years, even decades, without the disease becoming clinically evident.

Randomized Trials of Prostate Cancer Screening

There have been two large, prospective, randomized controlled trials of prostate cancer screening, one from the United States and the other from Europe. Preliminary reports from both trials were published in 2009. Given the controversy over screening since PSA testing became routine, the results of these two trials were highly anticipated.

The European Randomized Study of Screening for Prostate Cancer (ERSPC) enrolled 182,000 men in seven European countries from 1991 to 2003. This study concluded that PSA-based screening reduced prostate cancer mortality by 20%. This "positive" finding was balanced by the high rate of overdiagnosis and overtreatment. At a median follow-up of 9 years, the cumulative risk of prostate cancer was 8.2% and 4.8% in the control and screening groups, respectively. The absolute difference in prostate cancer mortality was 0.71 deaths per 1,000 men. This translated to the need to screen 1,410 men, and treat 48 of these men to prevent one death from prostate cancer. The authors noted that the number needed to screen is similar to that of mammographic screening for breast cancer. However, the positive predictive value of a positive PSA in this study was only 24%. As one might expect, metastatic disease (by bone scan) was found more frequently at the time of diagnosis in the control group (0.39 vs. 0.23 per 1,000 person-years). A greater proportion of diagnosed cancers were high-grade lesions (Gleason score of ≥ 7) in the control group, suggesting that many of the cancers found by screening were low-grade lesions. Benefits of screening did not appear to extend to patients 50–54 or older than 70. It is interesting to note that the average screening events during this 9–year period were only 2.1. This contrasts sharply with the current practice of yearly screening in the United States.[6]

At the same time, the initial results from the Prostate, Lung, Colorectal, and Ovarian (PLCO) Cancer Screening Trial was also reported. This U.S.-based study randomly assigned nearly 77,000 men from 1993 to 2001 to receive annual screening or usual care. This study was reported after 7 years of follow-up (earlier than initially planned). There was no difference in rates of death from prostate cancer between the two groups. The hazard ratio for prostate cancer diagnosis was 1.22 in the screening group. Median follow-up in the PLCO trial was 11.5 years, with presented data representing complete follow-up at 7 years. Advanced-stage (III and IV) disease was not seen more frequently in the control group, although there were more cases with Gleason scores of 8 and 9 (341 vs. 289). The overall rate of death from prostate cancer was low, with 94 total prostate cancer–related deaths occurring in the study population (50 in screening, 44 in control) at 7 years. This translated to two deaths per 10,000 person years in the screening group and 1.7 deaths per 10,000 person-years in the control group. Details on complications related to overdiagnosis and treatment are still being analyzed.[7]

Many significant differences could account for the discordant results seen between these two trials. In the ERSPC trial, biopsies were performed for any PSA level greater than 3, versus the current U.S. standard and PLCO cutoff of 4 ng/mL. The ERSPC was basically a collection of seven different trials, with recruitment and randomization procedures varying by country. Screening intervals in the ERSPC trial occurred predominantly every 4 years, although one center used 2-year intervals. This was based on an average lead time of 5 to 10 years seen in previous studies. The PLCO trial planned annual PSA testing for

6 years. In the PLCO trial, a significant proportion of men in the nonscreening arm had undergone PSA testing prior to enrollment in the trial (34% within the previous 3 years). Furthermore, because of the widespread use of PSA screening in the U.S., 52% of the patients in the control group had been screened by the sixth year of the study. This level of contamination certainly could have obscured the benefits of screening. The authors suggest that the cumulative death rate was low due to improvements in treatment and the number of patients who had undergone previous PSA testing. A lower death rate could have obscured differences as well.

There were, however, some similarities between the two trials. Both trials confirmed that screening detects more cases of prostate cancer, although the magnitude of this difference was more pronounced in the European study. Both trials evaluated men aged 55–74 years (ERSPC included patients 50–54 but focused on a core group of 55–69 years). These trials had a relatively short follow-up period for a disease with such a long natural history. In the ERSPC trial, the mortality rates between the groups began to diverge only after 7 or 8 years. The data safety monitoring board of the PLCO recommended that results be reported sooner than the planned 13-year follow-up, based on lack of benefit seen and potential harm(s) of continued PSA screening. The ERSPC trial was reported after its planned third interim analysis showed the above positive results; due to many prior interim analyses, that trial now has markedly reduced statistical power for future analyses. Regardless, there is no doubt that both trials will have updated results in the future.

Although these trials provide the best randomized controlled data on the efficacy of prostate cancer screening, the discordant results still leave room for controversy. Zealots will find justification from either study to continue supporting their views. In the end, the decision to screen an asymptomatic male for prostate cancer rests on the physician–patient relationship, and a frank and open discussion with the patient about the risks and benefits of screening, including the consequences of overdiagnosis and overtreatment, is warranted prior to the initiation of any prostate cancer screening test.

Summary of Guidelines

As mentioned previously, prostate cancer is the most common non–skin malignancy in men in the United States, with roughly 1 in 6 men affected in their lifetime. However, approximately only about 1 in 30 men will die from this disease. Thus, one common argument against screening for prostate cancer is the reality that many cases are clinically indolent and would never be found nor impact a man's mortality without screening. The harms attributable to screening are related to complications from biopsies as well as overdiagnosis. Overtreatment would account for the most significant adverse impacts of screening, as side effects related to prostatectomy, radiotherapy, and hormonal therapies are significant. Some would argue that the development of metastatic disease is both morbid and universally fatal, so if screening allows treatment at an earlier stage, it is worthwhile. Despite the available data, no consensus currently exists regarding the role of prostate cancer screening. However, widespread use of PSA testing continues. Few would disagree that, prior to PSA testing, a physician and patient should have a balanced discussion. Patients should be well informed regarding the PSA test's limitations (i.e., poor positive predictive value and imperfect negative predictive value) and the need for subsequent biopsies and procedures. Summaries of recommendations of various organizations are given in Table 3.1. Several decision-making aids are available to men to help make this decision. Some examples are given in Table 3.2. Well-informed men who value making the diagnosis early, even if this results in unnecessary treatment should undergo routine testing. Men at high risk (African American, first-degree family history) should also be given a recommendation to undergo testing. Men with life expectancies of less than 10 years would be likely to die of another disease, and thus screening is not recommended. For men at average risk for prostate cancer, the benefits of screening on prostate mortality remains a controversy, and thus the burden of deciding whether or not to screen falls to the individual patient and his physician.

Table 3.1 Summary of Various Recommendations

Organization	Recommendation	Year
American Cancer Society	In men whose life expectancy is >10 years, average-risk men should consider screening after a balanced discussion on risks vs. benefits after age 50. Men at high risk can start sooner. DRE is optional.	2010
American Urological Association	In men whose life expectancy is >10 years, a baseline PSA should be obtained at age 40. Future screening intervals based on this value. Screening should include both a PSA and DRE.	2009
U.S. Preventative Services Task Force	In men <age 75 years, the benefits of screening for prostate cancer are uncertain, and the balance of benefits and harms cannot be determined. Recommends against screening in men >75.	2008
National Comprehensive Cancer Network	Does not provide specific recommendations on whether screening should be offered or not, deferring to individual decision between patient and doctor.	2010

DRE, digital rectal exam; PSA, prostate-specific antigen

Table 3.2 Prostate Cancer Screening Decision Aids

Organization	Title	Web Address
Centers for Disease Control and Prevention	Prostate Cancer Screening: A Decision Guide	www.cdc.gov/cancer/prostate/pdf/prosguide.pdf
American Cancer Society	Should I be tested for prostate cancer?	www.cancer.org/prostatemd
Foundation for Informed Medical Decision Making	Is a PSA test right for you?	www.healthdialog.com
Mayo Clinic	Prostate cancer screening: Should you get a PSA test?	www.mayoclinic.com/health/prostate-cancer

References

1. Horner M, Ries L, Krapcho M, et al. SEER Cancer Statistics Review, 1975–2006. Bethesda, MD: National Cancer Institute, 2009. Available online at http://seer.cancer.gov/csr/1975_2006/index.html

2. Draisma G, Etzioni R, Tsodikov A, et al. Lead time and overdiagnosis in prostate-specific antigen screening: Importance of methods and context. *J Natl Cancer Inst* 2009;101(6):374–383.

3. DeVita VT, Hellman S, Rosenberg SA. Prostate cancer screening. In: *Cancer principles and practice of oncology*. Philadelphia: Lippincott Williams & Wilkins, 2005.

4. Ward E, Halpern M, Schrag N, et al. Association of insurance with cancer care utilization and outcomes. *CA Cancer J Clin* 2008;58(1):9–31.

5. Thompson IM, Pauler DK, Goodman PJ, et al. Prevalence of prostate cancer among men with a prostate-specific antigen level ≤4.0 ng per milliliter. *N Engl J Med* 2004;350(22):2239–2246.

6. Schroder FH, Hugosson J, Roobol MJ, et al. Screening and prostate-cancer mortality in a randomized European study. *N Engl J Med* 2009;360(13):1320–1328.

7. Andriole GL, Crawford ED, et al. Mortality results from a randomized prostate-cancer screening trial. *N Engl J Med* 2009;360(13):1310–1319.

Chapter 4

Clinical Presentation of Prostate Cancer

Hao G. Nguyen and Theresa Koppie

Symptoms and Signs

As noted in the previous chapters, prior to the prostate-specific antigen (PSA) era, physicians depended on the digital rectal examination (DRE) and clinical symptoms to detect prostate cancer. With the widespread use of PSA testing, prostate cancer at initial presentation has shifted toward earlier-stage disease, and patients no longer present with clinical symptoms or signs that would be apparent to the physician.[1] Today, detection of up to 80% of prostate cancers relies on a combination of DRE and PSA screening.

Since the majority of prostate cancers arise from the peripheral zone, symptoms are fairly rare during the early stages of disease. With increasing stage, prostate cancers can cause symptoms when they invade locally. Growth of the prostate into the bladder neck, urethra, or the trigone can cause irritative voiding symptoms such as urinary frequency, urgency, nocturia, and urge incontinence. Locally advanced prostate cancer can also cause obstructive symptoms such as hesitancy, intermittency, incomplete voiding, weak stream, or acute urinary obstruction. These symptoms are difficult to discern from those of benign prostatic hypertrophy (BPH), which is also common among aging men. Local invasion of prostate cancer into the ejaculatory ducts can result in decreased semen volume and/or the presence of blood in the ejaculate. On rare occasion, patients with locally advanced disease may present with erectile dysfunction as a result of cancer invasion beyond the prostatic capsule into the neurovascular bundle.

Because the ureters drain into the trigone near the bladder neck and prostate, local invasion of cancer into this region can result in bilateral or unilateral obstruction at the vesicoureteric junction. Such patients can present with acute renal failure or hydronephrosis and may require either internal ureteral stenting or percutaneous nephrostomy tube placement to relieve the obstruction.

Involvement of pelvic lymph nodes, resulting in the compression of the iliac veins, can lead to lower extremity edema. In rare occasions, nodal involvement can cause extrinsic compression of the ureters, leading to hydronephrosis and renal failure.

Metastatic prostate cancer can present with systemic symptoms such as anemia, renal failure, weight loss, bone pain, and back pain. Metastatic bone pain typically develops gradually, hence, specific questions should be aimed at eliciting the intensity, location, onset, and character over time. Spread to the lower vertebra can occur as a result of prostate cancer cells invading into Batson's plexus, a venous drainage between the pelvis and vertebral veins.[2] Spread to the axial and appendicular skeleton occurs by a hematogenous route, as these regions are extensively vascularized. Rarely, metastatic prostate cancer can result in retroperitoneal fibrosis, paraneoplastic syndromes, metabolic derangements, hypercoagulable states, generalized malaise, disseminated intravascular coagulation (DIC), constipation, nausea, and vomiting. Hypercalcemia from metastatic progression may produce neurologic, gastrointestinal, renal, and cardiovascular symptoms. The early and late symptoms and signs of prostate cancer are summarized in Table 4.1.

Indications for Prostate Biopsy

An abnormal DRE or elevated PSA may suggest prostate cancer; however, histologic confirmation is necessary for diagnosis of the disease. Transrectal ultrasound (TRUS)-guided prostate biopsies are indicated in men who have an abnormal DRE, an elevated PSA, or a prostate velocity (rising PSA level from test to test) of more than 0.35 ng/mL/year for men with PSA levels of less than 4 ng/mL or a PSA velocity more than 0.75ng/mL/year for men with PSA levels of 4 or more.[3–6] Table 4.2 lists the recommended indications for TRUS-guided prostate biopsy. The decision to proceed to prostate biopsy is based primarily on PSA and DRE; however, other important factors should be taken into consideration, including patient age, wishes, comorbidities, family history, ethnicity, and the number of previous biopsies performed. Patients of advanced age (>75 years) or with significant comorbidities (life expectancy <10 years) may not benefit from a biopsy (and subsequent treatment) for an elevated PSA alone. Patients who are younger, those with a significant family history of prostate cancer, and African American men are more likely to harbor prostate cancer when their PSA is elevated. Patients who have had high-quality (>10 cores) negative prostate biopsies in the past may be able to defer a repeat biopsy; but this decision should be made with their urologist. TRUS-guided biopsy should not be used as a screening test for prostate cancer due to its low predictive value.

Prior to recommending a prostate biopsy, every patient should be counseled on the potential impact of a prostate cancer diagnosis, including the often slow, untreated natural history of prostate cancer, as well as potential treatment options. Prostate cancer is ubiquitous among aging men. Autopsy studies have demonstrated that prostate cancer is present in 8% of men in their 20s, and increases to 80% among men in their 70s.[7] However, death from prostate cancer is low, at 224 per 100,000 men over 65 years old (0.002%).[7] In addition, patients should understand that a negative biopsy does not completely rule out a prostate cancer diagnosis, and that further PSA follow-up may be necessary. Table 4.3 summarizes management options based on TRUS-guided biopsy results.

Table 4.1 Symptoms and Signs of Prostate Cancer

Early Symptoms/Signs of Prostate Cancer	Late Symptoms/Signs of Prostate Cancer
Irritative voiding symptoms	Acute renal failure due to ureteral obstruction
Obstructive voiding symptoms	Erectile dysfunction
Urinary retention	Bone pain
Reduce ejaculatory volume	Back pain, pelvic pain
Hematuria	Paraplegia from spinal cord compression
Hematospermia	Lower extremities edema
Painful ejaculation	Anorexia, weight loss, and malaise
Flank pain, nausea due to hydronephrosis	Metabolic derangements

Table 4.2 Indication for Prostate Biopsy

PSA	DRE
PSA higher than age-specific range	Normal
PSA velocity: >0.35 ng/mL/year for PSA <4 ng/mL, PSA velocity >0.75 ng/mL/year for PSA >4 ng/mL	Normal
Any value of PSA	Abnormal
A low free PSA <10%, and consider if <25%	Normal
DRE, digital rectal exam; PSA, prostate-specific antigen	

Table 4.3 Prostate Biopsy Results and Management

Prostate biopsy results	Management
Negative or low-grade PIN	Annual DRE and PSA
High-grade PIN	Re-biopsy in 1–3 years
Atypical small acinar proliferation	Re-biopsy within 3 months
Prostate cancer	Work-up and treatment versus active surveillance
DRE, digital rectal exam; PIN, prostatic intraepithelial neoplasia; PSA, prostate-specific antigen	

Diagnostic Evaluation

Prostate Biopsy

With the increase of PSA screening starting in the 1980s, it is estimated as many as 800,000 biopsies are performed annually in the United States alone.[8] Prostate biopsies can be performed by either a transperineal or transrectal approach. However, the transrectal approach provides improved imaging and prostate sampling. The procedure is performed in the outpatient setting, with local anesthesia using a spring-loaded biopsy needle, joined to a transrectal ultrasound probe. The transrectal ultrasound allows real-time prostate imaging for template- or lesion-directed needle guidance biopsy. Since most contemporary prostate cancers cannot be seen on prostate biopsy, when a patient meets criteria for a prostate biopsy, the biopsy should be performed regardless of whether a hypoechoic lesion can be visualized at the time of the procedure. At the time of the procedure, the prostate can also be measured for treatment planning, and any significant anatomical variations can be noted.

To improve prostate sampling, variations in the prostate biopsy templates have been explored. Initially, sextant biopsies were recommended, with a sensitivity of 70%–80%.[9] Over the past decade, the number of recommended biopsy cores has increased from 8 to 12, and contemporary templates now include laterally directed biopsies, which sample the posterior and anterior horns of the peripheral zone. This approach has become the new standard of care, as more extended and laterally directed biopsy templates have been shown to significantly increase prostate cancer detection rates by 15%–30% and decrease the false-negative rate of prostate biopsy from 20% to 5%.[10,11]

Significant complications are uncommon after the TRUS-guided biopsy procedure. Low-grade side effects are common and self-limiting, including hematuria (15%–40%), hematospermia (36%), and rectal bleeding (2.3%–15%). More serious complications are less common and include urinary retention (0.8%–1.2%), fevers (1%–5%), and urosepsis (<0.6%).[12–14]

Imaging Studies

With stage migration toward lower-stage, lower-volume disease, imaging studies including TRUS, computed tomography/magnetic resonance imaging (CT/MRI), bone scan, or ProstaScint scan play a minor role in the management of early-stage prostate cancer. Instead, modern prediction tools that incorporate stage, grade, and PSA have replaced imaging studies in predicting the response to therapy. However, the imaging studies reviewed below may continue to play a role in the management of higher-volume or advanced prostate cancers.

Transrectal Ultrasound

Since the TRUS of the prostate was introduced in 1960s, TRUS has aided surgeons and radiologists in providing real-time imaging of the prostate during needle biopsy,[15,16] brachytherapy seed placement, prostate cryoablation, and high-intensity focused ultrasound (HIFU). Transrectal ultrasound can measure prostate volume with acceptable accuracy (within 10%).[17] When visible by ultrasound, prostate tumors generally appear hypoechoic compared with the peripheral zone of the prostate, but may be more difficult to identify in the transition zone of the prostate, which has varying echo texture.

The role of TRUS in diagnosing prostate cancer remains limited, with a wide range of sensitivity and specificity (50% to 92%).[18] With prostate cancer stage migration, fewer tumors that are detectable by TRUS (low sensitivity) are seen. Conversely, hypoechoic areas are frequently not cancerous on prostate biopsy (low specificity). In expert hands, TRUS may have a role in evaluating the extent of local disease and can aid in treatment planning. Extracapsular extension is suggested by a bulging or irregularity of the capsule in an area immediately adherent to a visible tumor nodule. Length of contact of a visible lesion with the capsule can also suggest microscopic extracapsular extension.

Computed tomography of the abdomen and pelvis plays no significant role in the diagnosis and local staging of low- and intermediate-risk prostate cancer due to poor prostate soft-tissue resolution, inability to distinguish benign from malignant nodules of the prostate, and poor visualization the prostatic capsule.[19–21] It may play a role in the evaluation of locally advanced disease, and in the evaluation of pelvic lymph nodes among patients at risk for nodal metastases. According to the National Comprehensive Cancer Network (NCCN) guidelines, CT scan is recommended to evaluate patients with clinical stage T3 and T4 prostate cancer, PSA of greater than 20 or a Gleason grade of 8 or more, or in high-risk prostate cancer suspicious of nodal involvement.[6]

Positron emission tomography (PET) relies on evidence of the increased cellular metabolism of the tumor cells, using ^{18}F-fluorodeoxyglucose (FDG) radiotracer. Because many prostate cancers possess low metabolic activity, FDG imaging does not optimally image local or advanced prostate cancer, and the results of FDG PET for prostate cancer have been disappointing (22,23). Furthermore, FDG is excreted by the kidneys into the urinary bladder, making disease within the prostate difficult to identify. With the development of new radiotracers (^{18}F-choline, ^{11}C-choline, and ^{11}C-acetate) that are capable of detecting the slow growth rate of prostate cancer, PET has a potential role in detecting recurrent prostate cancer after local treatment, as well as metastatic disease.[21]

Endorectal MRI is useful in local staging, specifically in detecting extracapsular extension (ECE) and seminal vesicle involvement, at a relatively high sensitivity and specificity.[15,21] Endorectal MRI differs from standard pelvic MRI in that it utilizes endorectal coils and a pelvic phased-array with a 1.5 or higher Tesla magnet. This provides a high-resolution, low signal-to-noise ratio image that is capable of distinguishing zonal anatomy as well as extension beyond the prostatic capsule. Previous studies found endorectal MRI to have a 91% sensitivity and 47% specificity in detecting ECE.[24] Another study reported a sensitivity of 95% and a specificity of 82% in diagnosing the presence of ECE in 73 patients.[25]

Identification of prostate cancers by endorectal MRI relies heavily on T2 weighted images, where cancers generally have decreased signal intensity when compared to the normal peripheral zone. Endorectal MRI is best performed at greater than 4 weeks after prostate biopsy, as post-biopsy hemorrhage can complicate tumor visualization. Choline compounds are elevated, and citrate compounds decreased in the setting of prostate cancer. Magnetic resonance spectroscopic imaging can improve the diagnostic power of endorectal MRI through the detection of choline, citrate, and creatine ratios within the prostate. Endorectal MRI is currently being used at select centers, and its role in urologic practice remains to be determined.

Bone Scan

Radionuclide bone scintigraphy (bone scan) with technetium[99m] has become the examination of choice for the detection of prostate cancer that has metastasized to the bone. Prostate cancer bone metastases start in the marrow and progressively destroy the bone by means of local cytokines that recruit and activate osteoclasts. Osteoclastic bone resorption results in an osteoblastic response. Bone scans can detect small osteoblastic and sclerotic changes in the bone, requiring only 10% change in bone mineral turnover for detection compared to plain films, which require 50% bone turnover. Bone scintigraphy has been shown by various studies to be highly sensitive and is currently viewed as the first-line modality in the detection of bone metastasis for prostate cancer patients.[26] It is particularly useful in determining the existence of metastatic disease in patients presenting with bone pain or elevated alkaline phosphatase. However, bone scintigraphy has poor specificity among asymptomatic patients, with frequent false-positive examinations due to degenerative disease and/or trauma. Selecting appropriate patients for bone scan can avoid unnecessary workups and excessive cost among low-risk patients. Previous studies have demonstrated a very low risk of bony metastasis, 0.6%, for patients with PSA levels of between 10.1 and 15 ng/mL and 2.6% for patients with PSA levels of between 15.1 and 20 ng/mL.[27,28] Patients with a Gleason grade of 8 or higher, a PSA level of 20 or more, or clinical stage T3 or higher should obtain a bone scan to determine whether they have local or distant disease, since the findings may alter their treatment plan. Of note, bone scintigraphy should be used judiciously when evaluating responses to therapy in advanced disease, due to the possibility of a "flare phenomenon," which is caused by an inflammatory response or increased turnover of hydroxyapatite and can be seen up to 3 months after systemic therapy initiation.[26]

ProstaScint® Scan

ProstaScint (^{111}In-capromab pendetide) is a monoclonal antibody to prostate-specific membrane antigen (PSMA) labeled with Indium (In 111) that can be used to localize sites of nodal or other soft-tissue metastasis. The test was rapidly approved by the U.S. Food and Drug Administration for use in detecting PSA-only recurrent disease after radical prostatectomy. However, several issues may limit its clinical utility. First, timing of imaging is important to optimize the signal-to-background ratio. The test requires a 4- to 5-day wait after infusion of radio-labeled monoclonal antibodies before a cross-sectional single photon emission computed tomography (SPECT) scan is performed, to allow for proper antibody binding, along with clearance of background tracer activity from the blood. To minimize problems with background signal, some institutions use subtraction techniques, in which red cells are counter-labeled with a separate tracer. Second, although the antibody has high specificity for PSMA, physiologically it recognizes an intracellular epitope of PMSA, which may only be exposed during conditions of cell lysis, such as cell death or destruction. The positive predictive value (PPV) of the ProstaScint scan is highly varied, from 11% to 66% in previous studies.[29,30] It also appears to have limited value in the setting of PSA failure after definitive local therapy.[31] The ProstaScint scan has not gained popularity due to limited clinical evidence, expanded use of risk-stratification models, and challenges in image interpretation; however, second-generation technology is currently in development.

References

1. Stephenson RA. Prostate cancer trends in the era of prostate-specific antigen. An update of incidence, mortality, and clinical factors from the SEER database. *Urol Clin North Am* 2002;29(1):173–181.

2. Thurairaja R, McFarlane J, Traill Z, et al. State-of-the-art approaches to detecting early bone metastasis in prostate cancer. *BJU Int* 2004;94(3):268–271.

3. National Comprehensive Cancer Network. Prostate cancer. NCCN clinical practice guidelines in oncology. *J Natl Compr Canc Netw* 2004;2(3): 224–248.

4. Scardino P. Update: NCCN prostate cancer Clinical Practice Guidelines. *J Natl Compr Canc Netw* 2005;3 Suppl 1:S29–33.

5. Kawachi MH, Bahnson RR, et al. NCCN clinical practice guidelines in oncology: prostate cancer early detection. *J Natl Compr Canc Netw* 2010;8(2):240–262.

6. Mohler J, Bahnson RR, Barry M, et al. NCCN clinical practice guidelines in oncology: prostate cancer. *J Natl Compr Canc Netw* 2010;8(2):162–200.

7. Sakr WA, Grignon DJ, Haas GP, et al. Age and racial distribution of prostatic intraepithelial neoplasia. *Eur Urol* 1996;30(2):138–144.

8. Halpern EJ, Strup SE. Using gray-scale and color and power Doppler sonography to detect prostatic cancer. *AJR Am J Roentgenol* 2000;174(3):623–627.

9. Roehl KA, Antenor JA, Catalona WJ. Serial biopsy results in prostate cancer screening study. *J Urol* 2002;167(6):2435–2439.

10. Presti JC, Jr., Chang JJ, Bhargava V, et al. The optimal systematic prostate biopsy scheme should include 8 rather than 6 biopsies: results of a prospective clinical trial. *J Urol* 2000;163(1):163–166.

11. Gore JL, Shariat SF, Miles BJ, et al. Optimal combinations of systematic sextant and laterally directed biopsies for the detection of prostate cancer. *J Urol* 2001;165(5):1554–1559.

12. Berger AP, Gozzi C, Steiner H, et al. Complication rate of transrectal ultrasound guided prostate biopsy: A comparison among 3 protocols with 6, 10 and 15 cores. *J Urol* 2004;171(4):1478–1480; discussion 1480–1471.

13. Ghan, KR, Patel U. Re: Complication rate of transrectal ultrasound guided prostate biopsy: a comparison among 3 protocols with 6, 10 and 15 cores. *J Urol* 2005;173(2):663–664.

14. Kakehi Y, Naito S. Complication rates of ultrasound-guided prostate biopsy: A nation-wide survey in Japan. *Int J Urol* 2008;15(4):319–321.

15. Purohit RS, Shinohara K, Meng MV, et al. Imaging clinically localized prostate cancer. *Urol Clin North Am* 2003;30(2):279–293.

16. Lavoipierre AM. Transrectal ultrasound and prostate-specific antigen in prostate cancer. *J Med Imaging Radiat Oncol* 2008;52(5):530.

17. Terris MK, Stamey TA. Determination of prostate volume by transrectal ultrasound. *J Urol* 1991;145(5):984–987.

18. Clements R. The role of transrectal ultrasound in diagnosing prostate cancer. *Curr Urol Rep* 2002;3(3):194–200.

19. Maio A, Rifkin MD. Magnetic resonance imaging of prostate cancer: update. *Top Magn Reson Imaging* 1995;7(1):54–68.

20. Brassell SA, Rosner IL, Mcleod DG. Update on magnetic resonance imaging, ProstaScint, and novel imaging in prostate cancer. *Curr Opin Urol* 2005;15(3):163–166.

21. Bouchelouche K, Turkbey B, Choyk B, et al. Imaging prostate cancer: an update on positron emission tomography and magnetic resonance imaging. *Curr Urol Rep* 2010;11(3):180–190.

22. Effert PJ, Bares R, Handt S, et al. Metabolic imaging of untreated prostate cancer by positron emission tomography with 18fluorine-labeled deoxyglucose. *J Urol* 1996;155(3):994–998.

23. Hofer C, Laubenbacher C, Block T, et al. Fluorine-18–fluorodeoxyglucose positron emission tomography is useless for the detection of local recurrence after radical prostatectomy. *Eur Urol* 1999;36(1):31–35.

24. Presti JC, Jr., Hricak H, Narayan PA, et al. Local staging of prostatic carcinoma: Comparison of transrectal sonography and endorectal MR imaging. *AJR Am J Roentgenol* 1996;166(1):103–108.

25. Flanigan RC, McKay TC, Olson M, et al. Limited efficacy of preoperative computed tomographic scanning for the evaluation of lymph node metastasis in patients before radical prostatectomy. *Urology* 1996;48(3):428–432.

26. Messiou C, Cook G, deSouza NM, et al. Imaging metastatic bone disease from carcinoma of the prostate. *Br J Cancer* 2009;101(8):1225–1232.

27. Lee CT, Oesterling JE. Using prostate-specific antigen to eliminate the staging radionuclide bone scan. *Urol Clin North Am* 1997;24(2):389–394.

28. Dotan ZA, Bianco FJ, Jr., Rabbani F, et al. Pattern of prostate-specific antigen (PSA) failure dictates the probability of a positive bone scan in patients with an increasing PSA after radical prostatectomy. *J Clin Oncol* 2005;23(9):1962–1968.

29. Taneja SS. ProstaScint(R) scan: Contemporary use in clinical practice. *Rev Urol* 2004;6 Suppl 10:S19–28.

30. Nagda SN, Mohideen N, Lo SS, et al. Long-term follow-up of 111In-capromab pendetide (ProstaScint) scan as pretreatment assessment in patients who undergo salvage radiotherapy for rising prostate-specific antigen after radical prostatectomy for prostate cancer. *Int J Radiat Oncol Biol Phys* 2007;67(3):834–840.

31. Thomas CT, Bradshaw PT, Pollock BH, et al. Indium-111–capromab pendetide radioimmunoscintigraphy and prognosis for durable biochemical response to salvage radiation therapy in men after failed prostatectomy. *J Clin Oncol* 2003;21(9):1715–1721.

Chapter 5

Pathology of Prostate Cancer

Regina Gandour Edwards

The prostate is an encapsulated fibromuscular and glandular organ located below the bladder and above the pelvic floor. It encompasses the posterior urethra and is penetrated by the ejaculatory ducts. It sits inferior to the bladder and lies contiguous with the bladder neck, where the seminal vesicles lie proximal to the gland. The prostate is bound by the urogenital diaphragm inferiorly and the levator ani laterally. It is separated from the rectum by a bilayer sheath known as Denonvilliers' fascia, and is held to the pubis by way of the puboprostatic ligaments. The prostate is covered by periprostatic fascia, which is comprised of two layers: the prostatic fascia, which surrounds the prostate, and levator fascia, which extends from the endopelvic fascia. Anteriorly, the endopelvic fascia condenses to form the puboprostatic ligaments. The dorsal venous complex is a network of veins that lies anterior to the prostate. The cavernous nerves responsible for erectile function course posterolateral to the prostate, between the prostatic and levator fascia.

Prostate (or prostatic) cancer is an adenocarcinoma (or "gland-forming" cancer) derived from the acinar cells of the prostate gland. Normal acinar glands are lined by an outer basal cell layer and inner secretory or luminal cell layer. The basal cells serve as a population of reserve cells to replenish the secretory cells. Current evidence suggests that molecular alterations to these basal cells promote carcinogenesis. Prostatic carcinoma cells show loss of this basal cell layer and are an important criteria in diagnosis (Fig. 5.1). The precursor lesion for prostate cancer is called *prostatic intraepithelial neoplasia*, or PIN. It is considered an epithelial malignancy but is still confined to the basement membrane. Prostatic intraepithelial neoplasia is analogous to other in-situ carcinomas such as ductal carcinoma in-situ (DCIS), the precursor to invasive breast cancer.

Pathologic Diagnosis of Prostate Cancer

Diagnostic material typically consists of multiple small-needle biopsy tissue cores representing a thorough sampling of the gland. The resulting tissue cores are

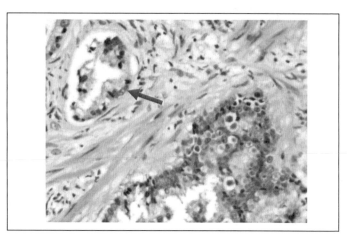

Figure 5.1 The large normal gland demonstrates an outer basal cell layer and inner secretory layer. The cancer gland has no basal cell layer (*blue arrow*) (See Color plate).

approximately 1 cm in length. Diagnosis is performed on standard hematoxylin and eosin (H&E) sections with application of the criteria for malignancy:

- Loss of basal cell layer
- Nuclear enlargement with nuclei
- Small, irregular glands with an infiltrating pattern

Frequently, focal areas of small acinar glands are identified that are inconclusive for malignancy because they lack definitive criteria. The utilization of a "triple stain" by immunohistochemistry may definitely document the presence or absence of a basal cell layer. Briefly, the triple stain includes two markers for basal cells: a low-molecular-weight cytokeratin cytoplasmic protein and a p63 nuclear marker. The third marker is α-methylacyl-CoA racemase (AMACR) an enzyme that has been demonstrated to be increased in prostate cancer cells. If both loss of basal cell layer and increased racemase is present in suspected glands, a diagnosis of prostate cancer can be made (Figs. 5.2 and 5.3).

Grading (Gleason's Scoring)

Once the diagnosis of carcinoma is made, the pathologist needs to accurately assess the grade of the prostate cancer. The grading system was developed by Dr. Donald Gleason, from his extensive observations of prostate cancer patterns correlated with patient outcome. The grading system has consistently shown excellent validity and usefulness as an independent factor for prognosis. The grading is based on the architecture of the cancer glands and consists of five grades, from 1 to 5, representing a decrease in differentiation. Thus, grade 5 is the least differentiated and is correlated with poorer patient prognosis.

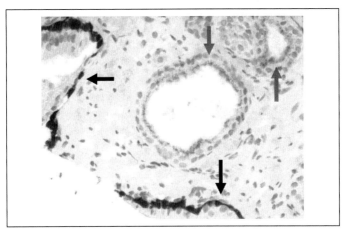

Figure 5.2 The large gland demonstrates an intact basal cell layer, with the presence of both cytoplasmic and nuclear dark brown staining (*black arrows*) and the absence of racemase (*red*). The cancer glands have an inverse pattern: no brown-staining basal cells and diffusely red staining cancer cells (*blue arrows*) (See Color plate).

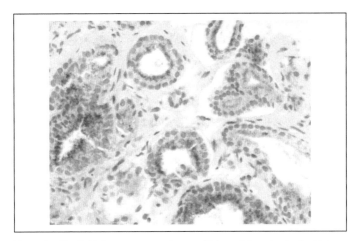

Figure 5.3 This field of prostate cancer shows multiple small, irregular glands with loss of basal cells and increased cytoplasmic expression of racemase (*red*) (See Color plate).

Within each grade multiple patterns of architecture are recognized, and typically more than one pattern is present in a diagnostic sample. The pathologist assigns two grades for a combined "score" (e.g., 3 + 5 = 8, 4 + 3 = 7), with the dominant grade listed first. The most common grade is 3, with the most common score being 3 + 3 = 6 (Figs. 5.4–5.7).

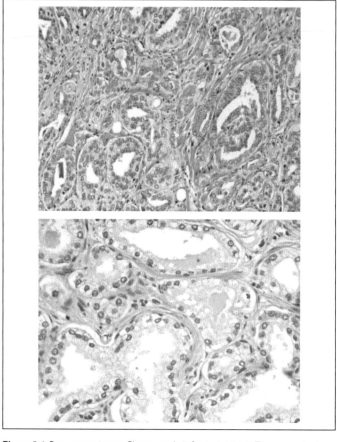

Figure 5.4 Prostate carcinoma, Gleason grade 3. Score: 3 + 3 = 6. The cancer glands are small and irregular but still individually defined (See Color plate).

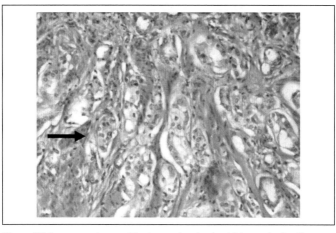

Figure 5.5 Prostate carcinoma with mixture of grades 4 and 3 (score: 4 + 3 = 7). Approximately half of the cancer glands are separate, but the rest are fusing together into nests with a so-called cribriform or "gland-within-gland" pattern (*black arrow*) (See Color plate).

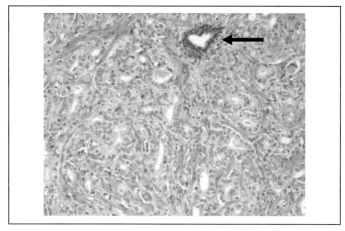

Figure 5.6 Prostate cancer with diffuse grade 4 glands. No separate glands are present. One benign gland is seen at the black arrow. Gleason score is 4 + 4 = 8 (See Color plate).

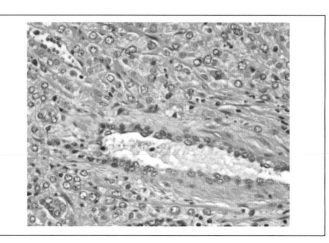

Figure 5.7 Prostate carcinoma with loss of glandular structure. The cells are in cords and sheets. This is grade 5 cancer with a single benign gland at the center of this image. Gleason score is 5 + 5 = 10 (See Color plate).

Pathologic Staging

True pathologic staging can only be performed on a radical prostatectomy specimen. Multiple sections are submitted to evaluate for the presence of capsular invasion, involvement of surgical margins, and involvement of the seminal vesicles (Figs. 5.8 and 5.9). Lymph node dissection is typically performed in the setting of a Gleason score of 7 or above on biopsy (Fig. 5.10).

Neuroendocrine Features in Prostate Cancer

Pure neuroendocrine carcinoma, as a small-cell carcinoma or carcinoid tumor, is uncommon. These tumors have features identical to neuroendocrine tumors in the lung. They lack prostate-specific antigen (PSA) and express neuroendocrine markers, such as synaptophysin. Neuroendocrine differentiation within a conventional prostate cancer is more common. Cells with eosinophilic granules are mixed with cancer cells that are reactive to neuroendocrine markers. The clinical significance of this remains uncertain.

Metastatic Carcinoma

Metastatic prostate cancer is largely detected by clinical studies including serum PSA and radiologic imaging. When indicated, tissue biopsy, including an immunohistochemical stain for PSA and/or prostate-specific acid phosphatase (PSAP), can be performed to confirm the diagnosis (Fig. 5.11).

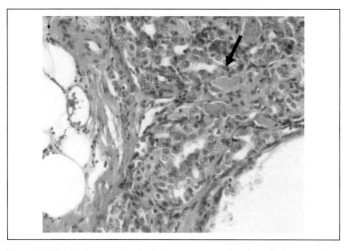

Figure 5.8 Section from capsule of radical prostatectomy showing multiple nests of prostatic carcinoma glands (*blue arrow*) adjacent to adipose tissue external to the capsule (See Color plate).

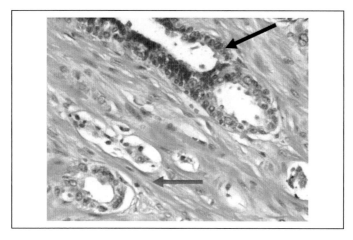

Figure 5.9 Section from the seminal vesicle showing cancer glands (*blue arrow*) adjacent to seminal vesicle epithelium (*black arrow*) (See Color plate).

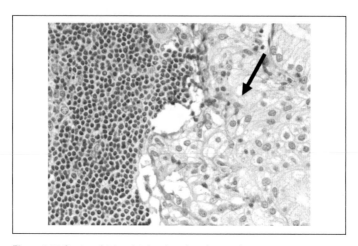

Figure 5.10 Section of right pelvic lymph node with nests of metastatic prostate carcinoma (*black arrow*). The large pink tumor cells contrast with the small blue round lymphocytes on the left (See Color plate).

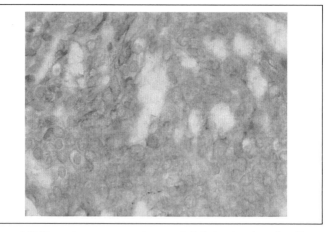

Figure 5.11 Metastatic prostate cancer in a supraclavicular lymph node confirmed by histopathologic evaluation. Immunohistochemistry demonstrates that the tumor cells are reacting to the brown Chromagen tagged to PSA. Note the diffuse brown staining of the cytoplasm in these cancer cells. This patient had a remote history of prostate cancer (See Color plate).

Suggested Reading

1. Eble J, Sauter G, Epstein J, Sesterham I, eds. *Tumors of the urinary system and male genital organs*. WHO Classification of Tumors. Geneva: IARC Press, 2004.

2. Epstein J. *Prostate biopsy interpretation*. Philadelphia: Lippincott Raven, 1995.

3. Amin M, Grignon D, Humphrey P, et al. *Gleason grading of prostate cancer*. Philadelphia: Lippincott Williams & Wilkins, 2004.

4. Epstein JI, Allsbrook WC, Amin MB, Egevad LL. The 2005 International Society of Urological Pathology (ISUP) Consensus conference on Gleason grading of prostatic carcinoma. *Am J Surg Pathol* 2005;29:1228–1242.

Chapter 6

Staging and Risk Stratification of Prostate Cancer

Jennifer Marie Suga and Primo N. Lara, Jr.

Prostate cancer staging at the time of diagnosis is critical to evaluate prognosis and to identify appropriate therapy for patients. Staging is based on the widely accepted American Joint Committee on Cancer (AJCC) Tumor-Node-Metastasis (T-N-M) *Classification for Adenocarcinoma of the Prostate*, seventh edition.[1] Primary tumor site (T) assesses the extent of involvement of the prostate gland and is based on clinical examination, imaging, endoscopy, biopsy, and biochemical testing. Nodal assessment (N) is necessary to evaluate the local regional lymph node involvement and is based on clinical examination or imaging. The metastases category (M) denotes distant spread of the tumor and is based on clinical examination, imaging, and biochemical tests (Table 6.1).

Clinical and Pathologic Staging

Clinical stage is determined using information obtained prior to initiation of definitive treatment. Physical examination of the prostate is an important component of the clinical stage. Those with a normal digital rectal examination (DRE) are considered to have T1 cancers. Cancers that are found incidentally while undergoing a transurethral resection of the prostate are T1a-b, with T1a tumors involving 5% or less of tissue resected and T1b tumors involving more than 5% of tissue resected. Those with a positive needle biopsy performed due to an elevated prostate-specific antigen (PSA) serum level alone are classified as T1c. T2 lesions are tumors confined within the prostate. T3 lesions extend through the prostate capsule and include seminal vesicle invasion, whereas in T4 lesions the tumor is fixed or invades adjacent structures.

Pathologic tumor staging uses the same information derived from diagnostic studies, supplemented by findings from surgical resection and pathologic evaluation of surgically removed specimens. Pathologic tumor staging for prostate cancer is similar to clinical staging, except that there are no T1 classifications. pT2 lesions are organ confined: pT2a refers to unilateral disease, involving one-half of one lobe or less, pT2b involves more than one-half of one lobe, and pT2c involves both lobes. pT3 denotes extraprostatic extension, whereas pT3a

Table 6.1 Prostate Cancer Staging: Tumor-Node-Metastasis (TNM) Definitions

Primary tumor (T)

TX: Primary tumor cannot be assessed

T0: No evidence of primary tumor

T1: Clinically inapparent tumor, not palpable nor visible by imaging

    T1a: Tumor incidental histologic finding in 5% or less of tissue resected

    T1b: Tumor incidental histologic finding in more than 5% of tissue resected

    T1c: Tumor identified by needle biopsy (e.g., because of elevated PSA)

T2: Tumor confined within prostate*

    T2a: Tumor involves 50% or less of one lobe

    T2b: Tumor involves more than 50% of one lobe but not both lobes

    T2c: Tumor involves both lobes

T3: Tumor extends through the prostate capsule**

    T3a: Extracapsular extension (unilateral or bilateral)

    T3b: Tumor invades seminal vesicle(s)

T4: Tumor is fixed or invades adjacent structures other than seminal vesicles: bladder neck, external sphincter, rectum, levator muscles, and/or pelvic wall

*Tumor that is found in one or both lobes by needle biopsy but is not palpable or reliably visible by imaging is classified as T1c.

** [Note: Invasion into the prostatic apex or into (but not beyond) the prostatic capsule is classified as T2 not T3.]

Regional lymph nodes (N)

NX: Regional lymph nodes were not assessed

N0: No regional lymph node metastasis

N1: Metastasis in regional lymph node(s)

Distant metastasis (M)*

MX: Distant metastasis cannot be assessed (not evaluated by any modality)

M0: No distant metastasis

M1: Distant metastasis

    M1a: Nonregional lymph node(s)

    M1b: Bone(s)

    M1c: Other site(s) with or without bone disease

* [Note: When more than one site of metastasis is present, the most advanced category (pM1c) is used.]

Histopathologic grade (G)

GX: Grade cannot be assessed

G1: Well differentiated (slight anaplasia) (Gleason score of 2–4)

G2: Moderately differentiated (moderate anaplasia) (Gleason score of 5–6)

G3–4: Poorly differentiated or undifferentiated (marked anaplasia) (Gleason score of 7–10)

includes microscopic bladder neck invasion, and pT3b involves seminal vesicle invasion. pT4 indicates invasion of adjacent structures, such as the rectum.

Regional lymph nodes are designated as N0 (no regional lymph nodes) and N1 (regional lymph nodes present). Regional lymph nodes can be either unilateral or bilateral, within the true pelvis, and below the common iliac artery bifurcation. Lymph nodes that are outside the true pelvis are considered metastases. Regional lymph nodes include the pelvic, hypogastric, obturator, internal and external iliac, and sacral lymph node groups.

Distant metastases are assessed as either M0 (no distant metastases) or M1 (distant metastases are present). M1a is a special designation for nonregional lymph node metastasis. These lymph nodes include the aortic, common iliac, inguinal, supraclavicular, cervical, scalene, and retroperitoneal lymph nodes. M1b is for metastasis to bone only, and M1c is for other sites of metastasis, excluding bone. Risk groupings for stage are summarized in Table 6.2.

Risk Stratification

It has been well established that pathologic Gleason score and pretreatment PSA are important components in assessing a patient's prognosis and in treatment planning. The AJCC cancer staging manual has recognized the importance of the Gleason score and PSA, and have incorporated these factors in identifying different prognostic groups. In addition to assessing the anatomic stage of the cancer, risk assessment models have been developed to estimate the probability of recurrence for a given patient. D'Amico et al. proposed a risk category system[2] that identifies patients into low-, intermediate-, and high-risk categories that predict biochemical recurrence after definitive treatment. These traditional categories were based on the 1992 AJCC clinical staging, PSA, and biopsy Gleason scores. This system provides a framework to assess the risk of biochemical recurrence after initial therapy. Low risk is defined as patients with stage T1c–T2a, a Gleason score of 6 or less or a PSA level of 10 ng/mL or lower. Low-risk patients have a less than 25% risk of recurrence after 5 years.

Table 6.2 American Joint Committee on Cancer (AJCC) Stage Groupings
Stage I
• T1a, N0, M0, G1
Stage II
• T1a, N0, M0, G2–4
• T1b, N0, M0, any G
• T1c, N0, M0, any G
• T1, N0, M0, any G
• T2, N0, M0, any G
Stage III
• T3, N0, M0, any G
Stage IV
• T4, N0, M0, any G
• Any T, N1, M0, any G
• Any T, any N, M1, any G

Patients with stage T2b disease, a Gleason score of 7, or a PSA level of between 10 and 20 ng/mL are deemed intermediate risk and have a 25%–50% risk of PSA failure at 5 years. High-risk disease is defined as patients with stage T2c or higher, a Gleason score of 8–10, or a PSA level of more than 20 ng/mL; patients with high-risk disease have a greater than 50% risk of recurrence at 5 years.

Clearly, there are those patients who initially present with low-risk disease but have prostate cancer with an inherently aggressive biology and are at higher risk for recurrence and mortality. Prostate-specific antigen velocity and doubling time have been studied to measure the potential aggressiveness of tumors. D'Amico observed that a PSA rise of more than 2 ng/mL/year prior to surgery was a poor prognostic predictor. These patients were found to have a 15% risk of death from prostate cancer within 7 years, whereas patients with a less than 2 ng/mL/year rise in PSA had a very low likelihood of morality.[3]

Prostate-specific antigen doubling time (PSA DT) has also been reported to be an important marker for aggressive disease. Klotz et al. looked at a cohort of 299 clinically low-risk patients and found that 24 patients who had a PSA DT of less than 2 years had a high rate of locally advanced disease at time of radical prostatectomy. Pathology results of these patients included 42% with pT2 disease, 58% with pT3a to pT3c disease, and 8% with N1 disease.[4] These data support the view that a short PSA DT is associated with highly aggressive disease.

Several other risk assessment tools have been published to predict outcomes for individual patients. For example, Partin et al. published probability tables that use a combination of PSA, clinical stage, and biopsy Gleason score to predict final pathological stage in localized prostate cancer. These tables were based on data gathered from 4,133 patients from three different institutions who had clinically localized prostate cancer and underwent radical prostatectomy. These probability tables can be used to inform patients on predicting ultimate pathologic stage.[5]

Kattan et al. developed a nomogram to predict the probability of treatment failure in 5 years for those who are undergoing radical prostatectomy for clinically localized prostate cancer.[6] These tools can be useful in counseling patients regarding the likelihood of recurrence for localized prostate cancer.

Overview of Treatment Options Based on Risk

In the initial evaluation of prostate cancer patients, it is important to keep in mind the life expectancy of the patient in the decision-making process regarding treatment recommendations. Life expectancy tables can be useful in counseling patients. In addition to considering overall life expectancy, the patient's overall health status must be carefully examined and incorporated into any treatment decisions. Comorbidities can influence a patient's outcome significantly. For example, in an unhealthy elderly patient with newly diagnosed prostate cancer, aggressive surgical treatment may be more harmful than a watchful waiting approach. Finally, patient preference should also be an important component in the treatment decision process, and careful education of patients regarding their various options is an essential part of a patient's initial evaluation.

Table 6.3 Risk-adapted Strategy Based on National Comprehensive Cancer Network (NCCN) Practice Guidelines in Oncology

Expected patient survival	Very low risk (T1c, GS <6, PSA <10, <3 biopsy cores +, <50% cancer in each core, PSA density <0.15 ng/mL/g)	Low risk (T1–T2a, GS <6, PSA <10)		Intermediate risk (T2b-T2c, GS 7, PSA 10–20)		High risk (T3a, GS 8–10, PSA >20)	Locally advanced (T3 b-T4)	Metastatic (Any T, N1, M0, or any T, N0, M1)
	<20 years	<10 years	>10 years	<10 years	>10 years			
AS	+	+	+	+	+			
Radiation Therapy-EBRT			+	+4	+4	+6	+6	+6,7
Radiation Therapy-IPBT			+	+/– 5	+/– 5			
Radical prostatectomy		+1,3	+1,3	+1,3	+1,3	+2,3	+2,3	
ADT							+	+

1 +/– Pelvic lymph node dissection if predicted probability of lymph node metastasis >2%

2 + Pelvic lymph node dissection

3 Followed by observation or RT if adverse pathologic features (positive margins, seminal vesicles invasion, extracapsular extension, or detectable PSA) or followed by ADT or observation based on lymph node metastasis

4 +/– Short-term ADT (4–6 mo)

5 In combination with EBRT only

6 + 2–3 years ADT

7 For any T, N1, M0 disease only

ADT, androgen deprivation therapy; EBRT, external beam radiation therapy; GS, Gleason score; IPBT, intraprostatic brachy therapy; PSA, prostate-specific antigen

Treatment recommendations should be tailored to each individual patient, based on the tumor characteristics, along with the patient's overall health factors. Acceptable treatment recommendations may include active surveillance, radical prostatectomy, or radiation therapy (either external beam radiotherapy or interstitial prostatic brachytherapy) for low-risk disease. These are discussed further in the next chapters. Intermediate-risk disease should be evaluated for appropriateness for active surveillance, radical prostatectomy, or radiation therapy, and also may benefit from additional androgen therapy deprivation. High-risk patients should be offered either radical prostatectomy or external beam radiotherapy, in combination with androgen therapy deprivation. Metastatic disease therapy should include primary androgen deprivation therapy, and in some selected patients, radiation therapy. A summary of NCCN practice guidelines in oncology (Table 6.3) is an example of one such risk-adapted strategy for prostate cancer treatment.

Conclusion

In the evaluation of a newly diagnosed patient, many factors, including extent of tumor; biochemical tests; pathologic features; patient characteristics, such as overall life expectancy and comorbid conditions; and patient preferences must all be taken into consideration to determine prognosis and make treatment recommendations. Men with localized prostate cancer have a wide variety of treatment options available to them, including active surveillance, external beam radiation therapy administered with or without hormone therapy, brachytherapy, and radical prostatectomy; these are discussed in more detail in subsequent chapters. Because no consensus currently exists regarding the optimal treatment for prostate cancer, patients and physicians are left with a challenging task of selecting a patient-tailored treatment that best suits individual disease characteristics, overall health, anatomy, and personal preferences. This decision-making process is hampered by the lack of randomized clinical trial data comparing cancer-specific outcomes, as well as the absence of standardized data comparing their side effects.

References

1. American Joint Committee on Cancer. *AJCC cancer staging manual*, 7th ed. New York: Springer, 2009.

2. D'Amico AV, Whittington R, Malkowicz SB, et al. Biochemical outcome after radical prostatectomy, external beam radiation therapy, or interstitial radiation therapy for clinically localized prostate cancer. *JAMA* 1998;280(11):969–974.

3. D'Amico AV, Chen MH, Roehl KA, et al. Preoperative PSA velocity and the risk of death from prostate cancer after radical prostatectomy. *N Engl J Med* 2004;351(2):125–135.

4. Klotz L. Active surveillance with selective delayed intervention: Using natural history to guide treatment in good risk prostate cancer. *J Urol* 2004;172(5 Pt 2): S48–50; discussion S50–51.

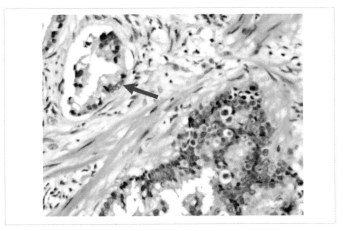

Figure 5.1 The large normal gland demonstrates an outer basal cell layer and inner secretory layer. The cancer gland has no basal cell layer (*blue arrow*).

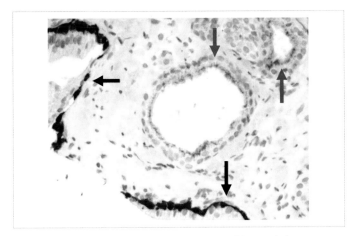

Figure 5.2 The large gland demonstrates an intact basal cell layer, with the presence of both cytoplasmic and nuclear dark brown staining (*black arrows*) and the absence of racemase (*red*). The cancer glands have an inverse pattern: no brown-staining basal cells and diffusely red staining cancer cells (*blue arrows*).

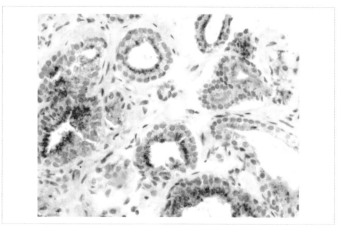

Figure 5.3 This field of prostate cancer shows multiple small, irregular glands with loss of basal cells and increased cytoplasmic expression of racemase (red).

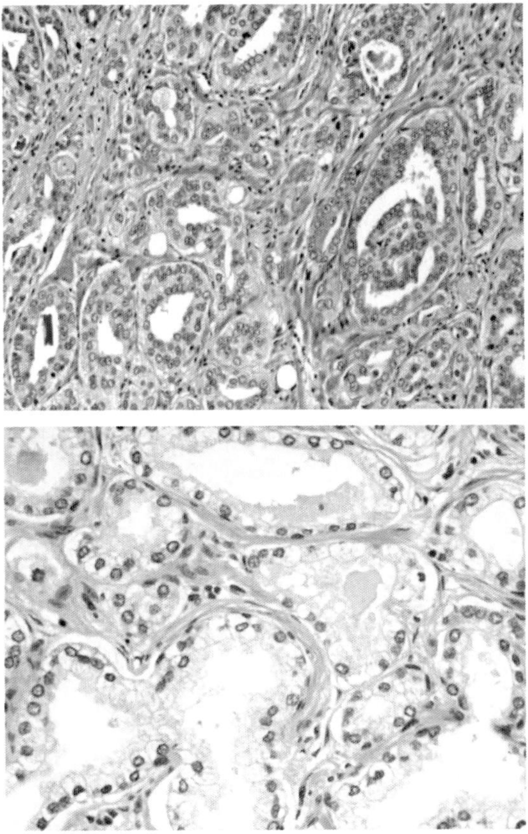

Figure 5.4 Prostate carcinoma, Gleason grade 3. Score: 3 + 3 = 6. The cancer glands are small and irregular but still individually defined.

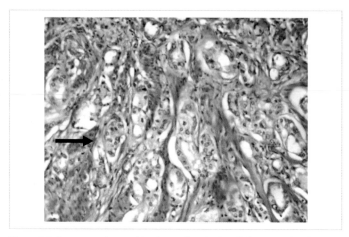

Figure 5.5 Prostate carcinoma with mixture of grades 4 and 3 (score: 4 + 3 = 7). Approximately half of the cancer glands are separate, but the rest are fusing together into nests with a so-called cribriform or "gland-within-gland" pattern (*black arrow*).

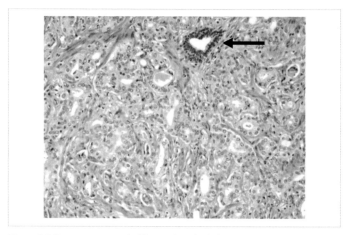

Figure 5.6 Prostate cancer with diffuse grade 4 glands. No separate glands are present. One benign gland is seen at the black arrow. Gleason score is 4 + 4 = 8.

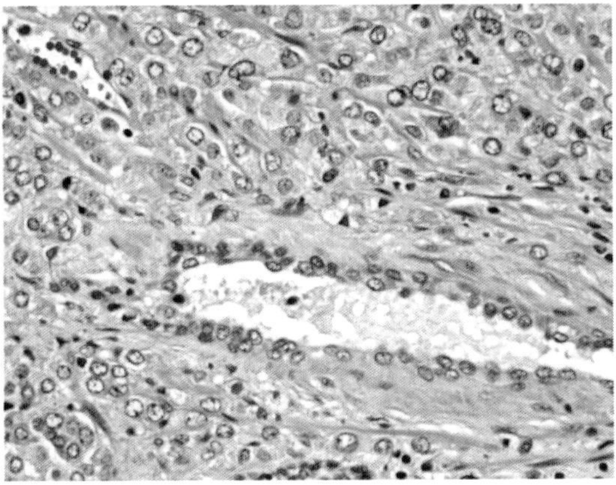

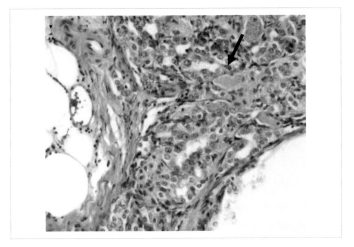

Figure 5.7 Prostate carcinoma with loss of glandular structure. The cells are in cords and sheets. This is grade 5 cancer with a single benign gland at the center of this image. Gleason score is 5 + 5 = 10.

Figure 5.8 Section from capsule of radical prostatectomy showing multiple nests of prostatic carcinoma glands (*blue arrow*) adjacent to adipose tissue external to the capsule.

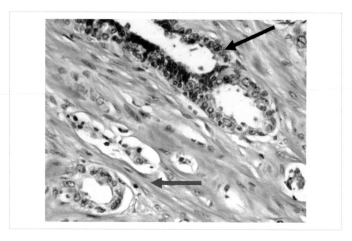

Figure 5.9 Section from the seminal vesicle showing cancer glands (*blue arrow*) adjacent to seminal vesicle epithelium (*black arrow*).

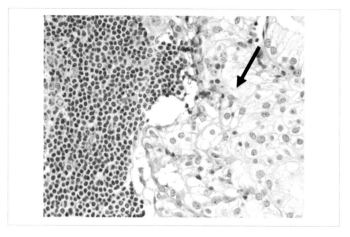

Figure 5.10 Section of right pelvic lymph node with nests of metastatic prostate carcinoma (*black arrow*). The large pink tumor cells contrast with the small blue round lymphocytes on the left.

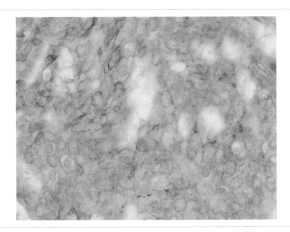

Figure 5.11 Metastatic prostate cancer in a supraclavicular lymph node confirmed by histopathologic evaluation. Immunohistochemistry demonstrates that the tumor cells are reacting to the brown Chromagen tagged to PSA. Note the diffuse brown staining of the cytoplasm in these cancer cells. This patient had a remote history of prostate cancer.

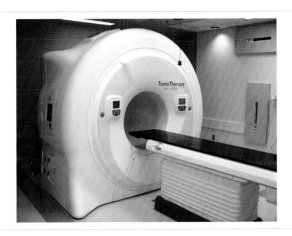

Figure 8.1 TomoTherapy Hi-Art System installed at the University of California, Davis. This system combines integrated computed tomography (CT) imaging with conformal radiation therapy to deliver sophisticated radiation treatments with precision while reducing radiation exposure to surrounding healthy tissue. In this system, a linear accelerator rotates on a ring-gantry. Intensity-modulated radiation therapy treatment is delivered while the couch is translated through the gantry bore in the same way as helical CT imaging is conducted. Photo courtesy of UC Davis Department of Radiation Oncology.

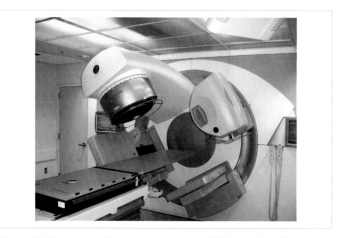

Figure 8.2 Elekta Synergy S installed at the University of California, Davis. Elekta Synergy S is a linear accelerator with 3D image guidance; it allows radiation oncologists to visualize tumor and normal tissue and their movement between fractions. This enables imaging of the patient in the treatment position prior to each fraction of radiation therapy, and delivery of radiation therapy to tumor while sparing normal tissue. Photo courtesy of UC Davis Department of Radiation Oncology.

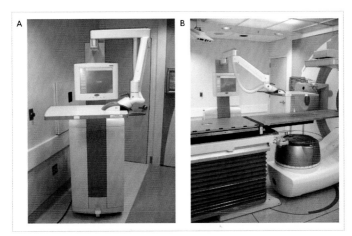

Figure 8.3 **A:** Calypso 4D Localization System for treating prostate cancer at the University of California, Davis. This technology works like a global positioning system (GPS). It determines the exact position and movement of the prostate during radiation therapy. Three tiny beacon electromagnetic transponders are implanted into the prostate in an outpatient procedure, similar to a biopsy. Each transponder is as small as a grain of rice. The beacon transponders in the prostate communicate with the Calypso 4D Localization System using safe radiofrequency waves. **B:** Calypso 4D Localization System and Elekta Synergy S linear accelerator ready for patient set-up and radiation therapy delivery. Photos courtesy of UC Davis Department of Radiation Oncology.

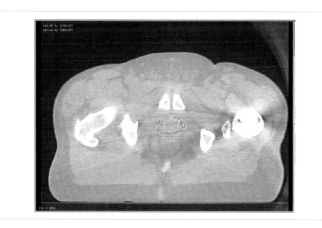

Figure 8.4 Post-treatment pelvic computed tomography (CT) scan of a 67-year-old man with a low-risk prostate cancer status post low-dose-rate (LDR) brachytherapy with [125]Iodine seed implantation. Note peripheral seed loading in the prostate, and isodose lines: 100% isodose line is in green and 150% isodose line is in blue. A radiation oncologist, urologist, and radiation oncology physicist perform the procedure in an operating room.

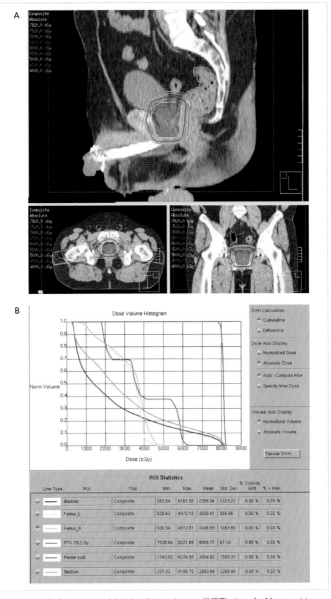

Figure 8.5A,B: Intensity-modulated radiation therapy (IMRT) plan of a 50-year-old man with intermediate-risk prostate cancer. He received 55.8 Gy in 1.8 Gy fractions to the prostate and proximal seminal vesicles, followed by boost to the prostate to a total dose of 79.2 Gy, along with 6 months of androgen deprivation therapy. The red area shows prostate with a treatment margin, the so-called the planning target volume (PTV). Thin lines around the PTV represent isodose distribution. Blue contour shows the bladder and orange contour the rectum.

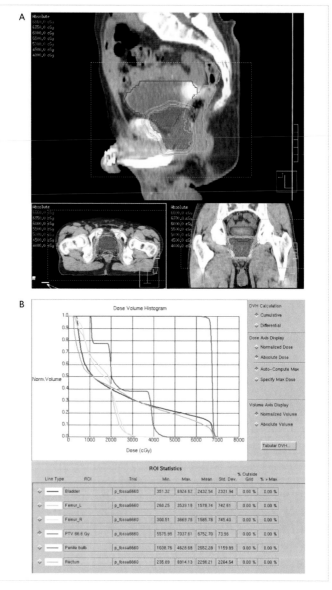

Figure 8.6A,B: Intensity-modulated radiation therapy (IMRT) plan of a 62-year-old man, who achieved undetectable PSA after prostatectomy, and a year later biochemical recurrence with a slowly rising PSA. He received 66.6 Gy in 1.8 Gy fractions to the prostate bed. The red area shows the prostate bed with a treatment margin to account for set-up error and motion. Note that treatment volume includes the vesicourethral anastomosis (right below the bladder), retrovesical space, and bladder neck—these are the most common locations of relapse in the prostate bed after radical prostatectomy.[37] Thin lines around the PTV show isodose distribution.

5. Partin AW, Kattan MW, Subong EN, et al. Combination of prostate-specific anti-gen, clinical stage, and Gleason score to predict pathological stage of localized prostate cancer. A multi-institutional update. *JAMA* 1997;277(18):1445–1451.

6. Kattan MW, Eastham JA, Stapleton AMF, et al. A preoperative nomogram for disease recurrence following radical prostatectomy for prostate cancer. *J Natl Cancer Inst* 1998;90(10):766–771.

Web Resources

Life expectancy tables   http://www.ssa.gov/OACT/STATS/table4c6.html.

Prostate cancer nomograms   http://www.mskcc.org/applications/nomograms/prostate/

Chapter 7

Surgical Treatment of Localized Prostate Cancer

Genevieve H. Von Thesling and Theresa Koppie

The radical prostatectomy (RP) was first introduced by Billroth in 1867 and was rapidly adopted by urologists in the 20th century. The operation saw significant improvements in the 1970s, and in 1982 was further refined by Walsh et al., after anatomical studies demonstrated the pathway of cavernous nerves responsible for erectile function.[1] The contemporary RP builds on years of surgical advances, resulting in a highly refined operation that is exquisitely sensitive to nuances of surgical technique. The goals of RP, in the order of importance, include cancer cure, urinary continence, and erectile function.

The salient benefit of RP is the potential for complete cancer cure due to the removal of the entire gland. Radical prostatectomy involves removal of the prostate, seminal vesicles, and the ampulla of the vas deferens while preserving the external urinary sphincter and, when possible, the cavernous nerves, which are responsible for urinary continence and erectile function, respectively. The RP can be performed in an open fashion through either a lower midline incision (radical retropubic prostatectomy, RRP), or through a perineal incision (perineal prostatectomy, RPP). Alternatively, the RP can be performed laparoscopically in the technique popularized by Guillonneau and Vallencien (LRP), or by robotic-assisted laparoscopic prostatectomy (RALP), an approach that is rapidly being adopted by urologists in the United States.

Lymph Node Dissection

The pelvic lymph node dissection (PLND) is often performed at the time of RP in an effort to capture potential metastasis and allow for accurate surgical staging. Although a variety of templates are used for PLND during radical prostatectomy, one common template includes all pelvic lymph nodes from the area bounded by the common iliac artery superiorly, the external iliac vein anteriorly, and through the obturator fossa to the circumflex iliac vein inferiorly.[2,3] Prostate cancer nomograms, described in the previous chapter, allow for preoperative prediction of the likelihood of lymph node involvement. [4,5] Currently, the National Comprehensive Cancer Network (NCCN) supports bilateral pelvic lymph node dissection for any patient with a 2% or greater risk of metastasis preoperatively.

Radical Retropubic Prostatectomy

Traditionally, RRP is the preferred approach for the majority of surgeons due to anatomic familiarity and ease of performing PLND. The nerve-sparing variation can also be performed through this approach and was characterized during open RRP.[1] This procedure offers a very low risk of rectal injury and offers excellent cancer control. Rates of positive surgical margins during RRP vary in the literature, ranging from 10% to 48%, with surgeon and institutional experience influencing these rates.[6,7] One multicenter cohort study of 7,756 patients undergoing RRP demonstrated a positive margin rate of 27%.[8]

Technique

The procedure requires a lower midline incision. The rectus musculature is separated and the space of Retzius is entered. If indicated, a bilateral lymph node dissection is performed. The endopelvic fascia is divided, and the space between the lateral prostate and levator ani musculature are bluntly dissected. The puboprostatic ligaments are incised where they attach to the prostate. The dorsal venous complex is oversewn distally and proximally, and incised. The lateral prostatic fascia is incised from the puboprostatic ligaments to the base of the prostate in order expose the prostate. The apical dissection is carried posteriorly to Denonvilliers' fascia. The neurovascular bundles are dissected from the prostate bilaterally. The urethra is incised, and the prostate reflected superiorly. The vascular pedicles to the prostate are clipped and cut. The seminal vesicles are identified and dissected free. The ampullae of the vasa deferentia are clipped and cut. The bladder neck is incised, and the prostate is sent for pathologic evaluation. The bladder neck is then everted and tightened if necessary. It is then anastomosed to the urethra via six absorbable sutures. Patients are usually discharged home on day 3, depending on procedure type, and typically go home with a urethral catheter in place, which is worn for 7–14 days.

Advantages

Most urologists are proficient at RRP. Pelvic lymph nodes are accessible for extended lymph node dissection, and complete removal of prostate and surrounding tissues is performed with minimal damage to adjacent structures.[9] RP has demonstrated less local progression, lower rates of distant metastasis, and improved overall and cancer-specific survival rates compared to watchful waiting alone.[10]

Disadvantages

Radical retropubic prostatectomy requires an abdominal incision, which is associated increased pain and prolonged recovery when compared to perineal or minimally invasive approaches.[11] Significant bleeding can occur and is generally higher than in laparoscopic approaches, due to the lack of tamponade provided by abdominal insufflation.[12,13]

Long-term Disease-specific Outcomes

The 10-year disease-specific survival after RRP ranges from 80% to 96%.[7,9] The 15-year freedom from PSA progression, as determined by two postoperative prostate-specific antigen (PSA) values of greater than 0.2 ng/mL, has been shown to be approximately 75%.[7] In a large series of 2,404 patients undergoing RRP at Johns Hopkins, the 15-year biochemical recurrence-free survival rate, when defined as a PSA of greater than 0.2 ng/mL, was 66%, and a 5-year metastasis-free survival rate was 82%.[9]

Complications

The overall early complication rate after RRP has been reported at approximately 10%–20%.[13–15] Thirty-day perioperative mortality is low, demonstrated at 0.0%–0.1% in two larger series.[14,16] Significant bleeding can occur with the procedure, ranging from 200 to 1,500 mL.[14,16,17] Deep vein thrombosis is a well-known complication after RRP, but occurs uncommonly, with 0.4%–1.6% of patients experiencing a thrombotic event after RRP.[16,17] Rectal injuries occur in less than 1% of patients and occur more commonly among patients who have had previous pelvic radiation, rectal surgery, or transurethral resection of the prostate.[14,18] Anastomotic stricture formation occurs late in approximately 1% of patients.[16]

Radical Perineal Prostatectomy

In general, less surgeon familiarity exists for radical perineal prostatectomy (RPP), and thus it is less commonly performed; however, data in the 1980s led to a renewed popularization for the procedure. The perineal prostatectomy is performed via the lithotomy position. It can be combined with a laparoscopic or open PLND as a separate procedure. Radical perineal prostatectomy is a good option for patients with low risk of metastasis who could possibly be spared PLND, and also for men with smaller prostates.

Technique

The patient is placed in an exaggerated lithotomy position. A curved Lowsley tractor is placed in the urethra, and its wings are opened intravesically to secure the prostate. A curvilinear incision is made in the perineum. The ischiorectal fossa is dissected bluntly, and the central tendon is taken. The anterior rectum is identified and the rectourethralis is taken close to the prostatic apex, where the rectum attaches to the perineal body. The plane between the rectum and prostate is then developed superiorly to the base of the prostate. Lateral dissection exposes neurovascular bundles, which are then dissected off of the prostate. The posterior urethra is incised, and the curved Lowsley retractor is exchanged for a straight Lowsley. The anterior urethra is incised, and the anterior prostate is dissected to the base. The anterior bladder neck is incised, and the Lowsley retractor is exchanged for a looped urethral catheter through the prostatic urethra for traction. The remainder of the bladder neck is incised. Vascular pedicles at the base of the prostate are cut and tied. The vasa deferentia and seminal vesicles are dissected free. If necessary, the bladder neck is reconstructed. The vesicourethral anastomosis is then sewn with interrupted absorbable sutures.

Advantages

Compared to RRP, in RPP, the anatomy may be more accessible in patients who are morbidly obese. The perineal incision is cosmetically more acceptable and is less painful than a lower midline incision.[19] Some surgeons report better visibility of the prostatic apex, allowing for easier anastomosis and improved continence, which approaches 95%.[20,21] This procedure is generally associated with shorter operative time, shorter recovery time, shorter hospital stay, and less blood loss than is RRP.[22]

Disadvantages

Radical perineal prostatectomy is, however, associated with a much higher rate of rectal injury (1%–11%) and fecal incontinence (5%–18%) than is RRP (21–23). Additionally, higher rates of capsular incisions and surgically induced positive margins have been seen compared to RRP.[24] Patients with low back or hip problems may not be able to tolerate this procedure.

Long-term Disease-specific Outcomes

Radical perineal prostatectomy has shown comparable long-term cancer control and similar positive margin rates as RRP.[22] Biochemical failure-free survival was 67% in a mean follow-up time of 24 months in one study.[24]

Complications

Capsular incisions and margin-positive rates are higher than in RRP.[24] In the Weldon et al. series, anastomotic stricture, inadvertent proctotomy, and venous thromboembolism were found to occur in approximately 1% of patients after RPP, with serious morbidity seen in 2% of patients. This same series reported zero perioperative deaths or mortality. Radical perineal prostatectomy is associated with a higher rate of rectal injury compared to other prostatectomy techniques. Rates of rectal injury have been reported as high as 11% in the literature.[21,22]

Laparoscopic Radical Prostatectomy

Laparoscopic radical prostatectomy was first introduced in 1997, and gained wider acceptance as outcomes data improved.[25,26] The procedure can be performed via transperitoneal or extraperitoneal approaches, the latter of which offers better protection and separation of adjacent abdominal structures at the cost of reduced operative space and maneuverability. Although there are no randomized data comparing open RRP to LRP, surgical success rates are generally similar.[26]

Technique

A Veress needle is placed carefully into the abdomen and the abdominal cavity is insufflated. A periumbilical port is placed through which the laparoscope is passed. Additional working ports are placed inferolaterally to the umbilical port. The pelvic lymph node dissection can be performed either before or after the prostatectomy, if indicated. A vertical incision is made in the cul-de-sac, between the bladder and rectum. Seminal vesicles are dissected free, and vasa deferentia is divided. A vertical incision is made through Denonvilliers' fascia, and the rectum is bluntly dissected downward. The space of Retzius is then opened by incising the urachus and performing a sharp or cautery dissection of the prevesical fat from the anterior abdominal wall down to the pubis. There, the endopelvic fascia is exposed and incised. The levator ani musculature is bluntly dissected from the prostate bilaterally. The dorsal venous complex is then either oversewn and incised or taken with a laparoscopic staple device. The bladder neck is then incised, and the vascular pedicles clipped and cut. The lateral fascia of the prostate are incised, and the neurovascular bundles are carefully dissected free from the prostate while minimizing electrocautery, in order to preserve cavernous nerve (erectile) function. The urethra is taken sharply, and the specimen is freed. A running urethral anastomosis is then performed. The prostate is removed through an expanded port site incision.

Advantages

Laparoscopic radical prostatectomy demonstrates shorter convalescence and less pain than does open surgery.[27] Less bleeding occurs with LRP, although there is no significant difference in transfusion rates between open and laparoscopic radical prostatectomy.[28] Laparoscopic radical prostatectomy can be performed at any center with laparoscopic capability.

Disadvantages

A steep learning curve is associated with LRP and therefore lengthy operative times and higher complication rates can be seen early in a surgeon's experience. Due to the technical challenges associated with mastery of LRP, this procedure should generally be performed at high-volume laparoscopic centers or centers with considerable surgeon experience. Rates of urinary leak, vascular injuries, and other organ injuries are higher than with open surgery.[26] Rates of rectal injury have ranged from 1.4% to 3.2% in the literature, and are generally slightly higher than for RRP.[26,29]

Long-term Disease-specific Outcomes

Data are limited by a lack of long-term experience with this technique. Short-term data demonstrate outcomes that are similar to open surgery. The 5-year PSA recurrence rate has been reported at 8.6%–18% after LRP.[12,30]

Complications

General operative complications are similar to those for RRP. Overall complication rates range from 10% to 22%.[26,31] Margin-positive rates range from 7% to 30%, but fall to lower values with greater experience.[12,29] Guillonneau et al. demonstrated conversion to open procedure was 1.2% and reported zero operative mortality. Deep venous thrombosis was seen in 0.3% of patients, and fistula and urologic organ injury were seen in up to 12% of patients. Blood loss has been shown to be less than with RRP.[29]

Robotic-assisted Laparoscopic Prostatectomy

The limitations and learning curve associated with LRP, coupled with advances in robotic technology, led to the popularity of RALP. The robot provides the same benefits as do other minimally invasive procedures but also offers improved 3D visualization and "wristed" technology, which could potentially lead to improved cancer resection, urinary continence, and erectile function.

Technique

The technique of RALP is the same as for LRP. Unlike LRP, in which the surgeon manipulates laparoscopic instruments at the bedside, with RALP, the camera and lateral working ports are occupied by robotic instruments that the surgeon manipulates remotely, while the assistant ports are used for retraction and suctioning by a bedside assistant. The primary surgeon is seated at the remote console several feet away. The remote console has dual eyepieces for 3D visualization, and houses controls that direct the robotic arms and laparoscope. The surgeon's thumb and index finger are inserted into control devices that allow the robot to precisely replicate human hand and wrist motion within the patient.

The first operative data was generated around 2002 and helped popularize the technique.[27,31] In general, RALP is found in the larger surgical centers, as there is a significant cost investment in robotic technology.

Advantages

Robotic-assisted laparoscopic prostatectomy shares all the advantages of LRP, but also offers improved visualization and "wristed" technology. 3D imaging with high magnification is valuable for viewing anatomic detail. These technical advances naturally replicate human movement; therefore, operative skills are more readily acquired by urologists. This may result in a more rapid learning curve and potentially improved outcomes.

Disadvantages

The disadvantages of RALP are similar to those of LRP. Robotic-assisted laparoscopic prostatectomy has a significant learning curve relative to RRP, although to a lesser degree than the purely laparoscopic approach.[27] The robot represents a considerable cost to a surgical center, and thus there are fewer centers that perform RALP.

Long-term Disease-specific outcomes

Data are too immature to draw concrete conclusions at this time. Early data suggest short-term cancer control rates similar to those of open technique.[13] Margin-positive rates are favorable, ranging from 9% to 15% in two larger studies.[28] Three-year follow-up after RALP demonstrates PSA recurrence rates similar to those of RPR, with approximately 93% disease-free.[32]

Complications

Complication rates are comparable between RRP and LRP. Like LRP, RALP is associated with shorter recovery time, shorter hospital stay, and less blood loss than is RRP.[27,28] The average hospital stay is 1 day after RALP, compared to 3 for RRP.[27,31] One small prospective study showed an average postoperative pain score of 4 versus 7 compared to RRP.[27] Improved operative time and positive surgical margin rates correlate with expanded experience.[31,33] Perioperative mortality is similar to LRP, and was reported to be 0.4% in one recent prospective study of 239 patients.[34]

Functional Outcomes

Urinary Function

There is no standard definition for urinary continence after radical prostatectomy, and various measures of continence have been utilized, including but not limited to physician-reported continence, patient-reported continence, quality-of-life questionnaires, and measurement of number of pads worn. Some urinary incontinence is almost universally noted in the immediate postoperative period. Symptoms generally resolve within 3–6 months of surgery, but infrequently persist for as long as 18 months or more. Kegel exercises are encouraged early in the postoperative period and contribute to regaining sphincter control. Studies reporting urinary incontinence rates after radical prostatectomy are generally single-center studies and vary in when and how continence is measured, thus the reported rates of urinary incontinence after RP varies widely, from 7% to 18% at 12 months. However, most centers of excellence report continence rates of less than 10%.[1,13,15,35] Incontinence rates according to surgery type are reported in Table 7.1.

Table 7.1 Reported Continence Rates by Procedure

RRP	RPP	LRP/MIRP[2]	RALP
>90% at 12 mo[1]. 93% pad-free at 12–18 mo. [15,35] 91.6% at 18 mo.[37] 95% at 24 mo.[7]	95% at 10 mo.[20]	90%–92% at 12 mo.[29] 82%–95%[12] 84.9% at 12 mo.[30] 81.8%[2,3,13]	92% at 6 mo.[31] 97% at 12 mo.[33]

[1]With preservation of external sphincter

[2]Minimally invasive radical prostatectomy (LRP & RALP)

[3]Endpoint unclear

RRP, radical retropubic prostatectomy; RPP, radical perineal prostatectomy; LRP, laparoscopic radical prostatectomy; RALP, robotic-assisted laparoscopic prostatectomy

Erectile Function

Erectile dysfunction is common after radical prostatectomy, ranging from 44% to 95%. Postoperative recovery of erectile function is highly age-dependent, with odds of success declining rapidly with advanced age.[36,37] Other critical factors in maintaining postoperative erectile function include patient preoperative erectile function, comorbid conditions such as cardiovascular disease or diabetes, and whether a nerve-sparing operation could be performed.[38] Early postoperative use of erectile function aids and penile rehabilitation are recommended to optimize erectile function.[39] To date, there is no standard definition of postprostatectomy potency, making erectile function rates difficult to interpret and compare. Potency rates by procedure are summarized in Table 7.2.

Rectal Function

Rectal dysfunction is uncommon after radical prostatectomy, but can be an important factor in treatment decision-making. Variations in rectal functional outcomes exist between RRP and RPP, as reported in Table 7.3, but also exist between surgery and radiation therapy, in which reported rates of rectal side effects range from 18% to 62%.[40,41]

Follow-up Strategies Postprostatectomy

The half-life of PSA is 3 days, thus the serum PSA should fall to undetectable levels within 3 to 4 weeks of RP. Prostate-specific antigen surveillance is generally performed every 3 to 6 months for 1 year, then every 6 months from the second through fifth years, then annually for 10 years. Currently, there is no standard definition for biochemical failure after RP. Because small amounts of PSA can represent benign glands at the surgical margin, low but detectable PSA levels may not indicate disease recurrence. Commonly used values that are currently used to indicate prostate cancer recurrence include PSA levels of 0.2 ng/mL or more, or 0.4 ng/mL or more.[42,43]

An abnormally elevated PSA after RP could represent either micrometastatic disease, locally recurrent disease, or the presence of residual benign prostate tissue. Determining the source of PSA is necessary for appropriate treatment planning; however, diagnostic modalities that can identify cancer in the curable range are limited. Currently, NCCN guidelines recommend that salvage (post-RP) radiation therapy be administered when the PSA remains below 2, and more recent data suggest that earlier salvage radiation therapy (<1 ng/mL) may result in superior recurrence-free survival.[42,44]

Prostate-specific antigen kinetics, pathologic stage, margin status, and Gleason score provide the best means of predicting the likelihood of local recurrence, which could potentially respond to salvage radiation therapy. Encouraging predictive factors include Gleason score of 7 or less, no lymph node or seminal vesicle invasion, PSA doubling time of greater than 6–10 months, PSA velocity of less than 0.75 ng/mL/yr, and PSA recurrence occurring at greater than 1–2 years after surgery.

Table 7.2 Reported Erectile Function Rates by Procedure (Preoperatively Potent Patients)

RRP	RPP	LRP/MIRP	RALP
50%–90%[1][35]	70% at 24 mo.[20]	52–78%[12]	81% at 12 mo.[33]
76%[1], 53%[3] at 18 mo.[15]		52.5%[4][30]	59% at 6 mo.[31]
34%[2], 41%[3], 44%[1] at 18 mo.[37]		66.2%[4,5][13]	
70% at 24 mo.[7]			

[1]Bilateral nerve-sparing

[2]Non nerve-sparing

[3]Unilateral nerve-sparing

[4]Varying endpoint

[5]Minimally invasive radical prostatectomy (MIRP)

RRP, radical retropubic prostatectomy; RPP, radical perineal prostatectomy; LRP, laparoscopic radical prostatectomy; RALP, robotic-assisted laparoscopic prostatectomy

Table 7.3 Reported Rectal Complication Rates by Procedure

	RRP	RPP
Fecal Incontinence	1%[29]	5–18%[21,23]
	5%[21]	

RRP, radical retropubic prostatectomy; RPP, radical perineal prostatectomy

Adjuvant Therapies Following Prostatectomy

Adjuvant radiation therapy has recently shown a potential benefit for patients with adverse pathologic features at the time of RP, such as positive surgical margins, extracapsular extension, and seminal vesicle invasion. Long-term results of two randomized clinical trials demonstrated improved biochemical recurrence and metastasis-free and overall survival for those patients who receive adjuvant radiation therapy after RP compared with RP alone.[45,46]

Hormone therapy should be considered for node-positive prostate cancer after RP and LND. Messing et al. showed significant improvements in overall survival (HR 1.84, p = .04), disease-specific survival (HR 4.09, p = 0.0004), and progression-free survival (HR 3.42, p <0.0001) at a median of 11.9 years among men who received immediate hormonal therapy when compared with those who received deferred treatment.[47]

Other Surgical Options

Cryosurgical Ablation of the Prostate

Cryotherapy is a minimally invasive treatment option for the management of prostate cancer. In this procedure, cryotherapy probes are placed into the prostate under transrectal ultrasound guidance. A urethral warmer protects the periurethral tissues as liquid nitrogen or pressurized gases are circulated through the cryotherapy probes. This induces freeze–thaw cycles to optimal temperatures of –40° to –50°C, resulting in injury at the cellular level, including mechanical and osmotic shock and cellular hypoxia. Real-time ultrasound imaging assures that the ice ball extends beyond the limits of the tumor.

Long et al. performed a multi-institutional analysis of 975 contemporary patients who underwent cryotherapy as primary therapy for prostate cancer.[48] Of those patients who were treated with a second-generation cryotherapy device, the 5-year freedom from biochemical recurrence (PSA >1 ng/mL) was 76%. Erectile dysfunction was common at 93%. Urinary incontinence was noted in 7.5% of patients. Rectourethral fistula occurred in 0.5% of patients. Salvage cryotherapy may also be an option for patients with radio-recurrent prostate cancer, with contemporary PSA recurrence-free survival rates ranging from 31% to 51%.[48]

High-intensity Focused Ultrasound

High-intensity focused ultrasound (HIFU) uses focused ultrasound applied through a transrectal probe to generate temperatures in the prostate up to 100°C. This heat ablates prostate cancer through coagulation, cavitation bubbles, and coagulative necrosis. Early studies report a short-term progression-free survival rate of 70% (post-treatment positive biopsy or a PSA >0.4 ng/mL). Side effects include urinary retention in 20% of patients and erectile dysfunction in 27%–61%.[49,50] High-intensity focused ultrasound is currently under investigation as a primary treatment for prostate cancer.

References

1. Walsh PC, Donker PJ. Impotence following radical prostatectomy: Insight into etiology and prevention. *J Urol* 1982;128(3):492–497.

2. Wein AJ, Kavoussi LR, Novick AC, et al. *Campbell-Walsh urology*, 9th ed., Chapter 95. Philadelphia: Saunders, 2007.

3. Studer UE. Should pelvic lymph node dissection be performed with radical prostatectomy? Yes. *J Urol* 2010;183(4):1285–1287.

4. Partin AW, Mangold LA, Lamm DM, et al. Contemporary updated of prostate cancer staging nomograms (Partin tables) for the new millennium. *Urology* 2001;58(6):843–848.

5. Kattan MW, Eastham JA, Wheeler TM, et al. Counseling men with prostate cancer: A nomogram for predicting the presence of small, moderately differentiated, confined tumors. *J Urol* 2003;170(5):1792–1797.

6. Eastham JA, Kattan MW, Riedel E, et al. Variations among individual surgeons in the rate of positive surgical margins in radical prostatectomy specimens. *J Urol* 2003;170(6):2292–2295.

7. Bianco FJ, Scardino PT, Eastham JA. Radical prostatectomy: Long-term cancer control and recovery of sexual and urinary function ("trifecta"). *Urology* 2005;66:83–94.

8. Vickers A, Bianco F, Cronin A, et al. The learning curve for surgical margins after open radical prostatectomy: Implications for margin status as an oncological end point. *J Urol* 2010;183(4):1360–1365.

9. Han M, Partin AW, Pound CR, et al. Long-term biochemical disease free and cancer specific survival following anatomic radical retropubic prostatectomy: the 15 year Johns Hopkins experience. *Urol Clin North Am* 2001;28(3):555–565.

10. Bill-Axelson A, Holmberg L, Ruutu M, et al. Radical prostatectomy versus watchful waiting in early prostate cancer. *N Engl J Med* 2005;352:1977–1984.

11. Hedican SP, Walsh PC. Postoperative bleeding following radical retropubic prostatectomy. *J Urol* 1994;152:1181–1183.

12. Romero-Otero J, Touijer K, Guillonneau B. Laparoscopic radical prostatectomy: Contemporary comparison with open surgery. *Urol Oncol* 2007;25(6):499–504.

13. Hu JC, Xiangmei G, Lipsitz S, et al. Comparative effectiveness of minimally invasive vs. open radical prostatectomy. *JAMA* 2009;302(14):1557–1564.

14. Catalona WJ, Carvalhal GF, Mager DE, Smith DS. Potency, continence and complication rates in 1,870 consecutive radical retropubic prostatectomies. *J Urol* 1999;162(2):433–438.

15. Kundu SD, Roehl KA, Eggener SE, et al. Potency, continence and complications in 3,477 consecutive radical retropubic prostatectomies. *J Urol* 2004;172(6):2227–2231.

16. Lepor H, Neider AM, Ferrandino MN. Intraoperative and postoperative complications of radical retropubic prostatectomy in a consecutive series of 1,000 cases. *J Urol* 2001;166:1729–1733.

17. Zerbib M, Zelefsky MJ, Celestia SH, Peter RC. Conventional treatments of localized prostate cancer. *Urology* 2008;72(6 Sup):S25–35.

18. McLaren RH, Barrett DM, Zincke H. Rectal injury occurring at radical retropubic prostatectomy for prostate cancer: Etiology and treatment. *Urology* 1993;42(4):401–405.

19. Korman HJ, Harris MJ, Dyche DJ. Prostate cancer: Radical perineal prostatectomy. *Emedicine Urology* 2009. Available online at emedicine.medscape.com.

20. Weldon VE, Tavel FR, Neuwirth H. Continence, potency and morbidity after radical perineal prostatectomy. *J Urol* 1997;158(4):1476.

21. Bishoff JT, Motley G, Optenberg SA, et al. Incidence of fecal and urinary incontinence following radical perineal and retropubic prostatectomy in a national population. *J Urol* 1998;160(2):454–458.

22. Janoff DM, Parra RO. Contemporary appraisal of radical perineal prostatectomy. *J Urol* 2005;173(6):1863–1870.

23. Kirschner-Hermanns R, Borchers H, Reineke T, et al. Fecal incontinence after radical perineal prostatectomy: A prospective study. *Urology* 2005;65(2):337–342.

24. Boccon-Gimod L, Ravery V, Vordos D, et al. Radical prostatectomy for prostate cancer: The perineal approach increases the risk of surgically induced positive margins and capsular incisions. *J Urol* 1998;160(4): 1383–1385.

25. Schuessler WW, Schulam PG, Clayman RV, Kavoussi LR. Laparoscopic radical prostatectomy: Initial short-term experience. *Urology* 1997;50(6):854–857.

26. Guillonneau B, Rozet F, Cathelineau X, et al. Perioperative complications of laparoscopic radical prostatectomy: The Monsouris 3-year experience. *J Urol* 2002;167(1):51–56.

27. Menon M, Tewari A, Baize B, et al. Prospective comparison of radical retropubic prostatectomy and robot-assisted anatomic prostatectomy: The Vattikuti Urology Institute experience. *Urology* 2002;60(5):864–868.

28. Tewari A, Srivasatava A, Menon M. A prospective comparison of radical retropubic and robot-assisted prostatectomy: Experience in one institution. *BJU* 2003;92(3):205–210.

29. Rassweiler J, Seemann O, Schulze M, et al. Laparoscopic versus open radical prostatectomy: A comparative study at a single institution. *J Urol* 2003;169(5): 1689–1693.

30. Rassweiler J, Stolzenburg J, Sulser T, et al. Laparoscopic radical prostatectomy—the experience of the German Laparoscopic Working Group. *Eur Urol* 2006;49(1):113–119.

31. Menon M, Tewari A, Peabody JO, et al. Vattikuti Institute prostatectomy, a technique of robotic radical prostatectomy for management of localized carcinoma of the prostate: Experience of over 1100 cases. *Urol Clin North Am* 2004;31(4):701–717.

32. Krambeck AE, DiMarco DS, Rangel LJ, et al. Radical prostatectomy for prostatic adenocarcinoma: A matched comparison of open retropubic and robot-assisted techniques. *BJU* 2009;103(4):448–453.

33. Ficarra V, Novara G, Secco S, et al. Predictors of positive surgical margins after laparoscopic robot assisted radical prostatectomy. *J Urol* 2009;182(6):2682–2688.

34. Lasser MS, Renzulli J, Turini GA, et al. An unbiased prospective report of perioperative complications of robot-assisted laparoscopic radical prostatectomy. *Urology* 2010;75(5):1083–1089.

35. Walsh PC. Patient reported urinary continence and sexual function after anatomic radical prostatectomy. *J Urol* 2000;164(1):242.

36. National Comprehensive Cancer Network. NCCN clinical practice guidelines in oncology: Prostate cancer, 2010. Available online at http//:nccn.org

37. Stanford JL, Feng Z, Hamilton AS, et al. Urinary and sexual function after radical prostatectomy for clinically localized prostate cancer: The Prostate Cancer Outcomes study. *JAMA* 2000;283(3):354–360.

38. Hollenbeck BK, Dunn RL, Wei JT, et al. Determinants of long-term sexual health outcome after radical prostatectomy measured by a validated instrument. *J Urol* 2003;169:1453–1457.

39. Mulhall JP, Morgentaler A. Penile rehabilitation should become the norm for radical prostatectomy patients. *JSM* 2007;4(3):538–543.

40. Theodorescu D, Gillenwater JY, Koutrouvelis PG. Prostatourethral-rectal fistula after prostate brachytherapy. *Cancer* 2000: 89:2085–2091.

41. Lesperance RN, Kjorstadt RJ, Halligan JB, Steele SR. Colorectal complications of external beam radiation versus brachytherapy for prostate cancer. *Am J Surg* 2007;195(5):616–620.

42. Amling CL, Bergstrahl EJ, Blute ML, et al. Defining prostate specific antigen progression after radical prostatectomy: What is the most appropriate cut point? *J Urol* 2001;166(6):2321–2322.

43. Stephenson AJ, Kattan MW, Eastham JA, et al. Defining biochemical recurrence of prostate cancer after radical prostatectomy: A proposal for a standardized definition. *J Clin Oncol* 2006;24(24):3973–3978.

44. Gretzer MB, Trock BJ, Han M, Walsh PC. A critical analysis of the interpretation of biochemical failure in surgically treated patients using the American Society for Therapeutic Radiation and Oncology Criteria. *J Urol* 2002;168(4):1419–1422.

45. Van der Kwast TH, Collette L, Bolla M. Adjuvant radiotherapy after surgery for pathologically advanced prostate cancer. *J Clin Oncol* 2007;25(10):5671–5672.

46. Thompson IM, Tangen CM, Paradelo J, et al. Adjuvant radiotherapy for pathological T3N0M0 prostate cancer significantly reduces risk of metastases and improves survival: Long-term follow-up of a randomized clinical trial. *J Urol* 2009;181(3):956–962.

47. Messing EM, Manola J, Yao J, et al. Immediate versus deferred androgen deprivation treatment in patients with node-positive prostate cancer after radical prostatectomy and pelvic lymphadenectomy. *Lancet Oncol* 2006;7(6):472–479.

48. Long JP, Bahn D, Lee F, et al. Five-year retrospective, multi-institutional pooled analysis of cancer-related outcomes after cryosurgical ablation of the prostate. *Urology* 2001;57(3):518–523.

49. Blana A, Walter B, Rogenhofer S, Wieland WF. High-intensity focused ultrasound for the treatment of localized prostate cancer: 5-year experience. *Urology* 2004;63(2):297–300.

50. Pickles T, Goldenberg L, Steinhoff G. Technology review: High intensity focused ultrasound for prostate cancer. *Can J Urol* 2005;12(2):2593–2597.

Chapter 8

Treatment of Localized Prostate Cancer: Radiation Therapy

Sinisa Stanic and Richard K. Valicenti

Overview of Radiation Therapy Biology

External beam radiotherapy employs high-energy photons, typically 6–10 MV. The biologic damage is caused by direct and indirect action of the photons. With direct action, a secondary electron resulting from absorption of a high-energy photon interacts with DNA to produce an effect, whereas with indirect action, the secondary electron interacts with a water molecule to generate a hydroxyl radical, producing DNA damage. More than 60% of the biological damage is caused by indirect action. There is a good correlation between cancer cells killed and cells with dicentric and ring chromosomes.[1] This means that the nucleus of the cell, specifically the DNA, is the principal target of radiation.

Following exposure to radiation, cancer cells may die attempting the next mitosis (mitotic death) or through programmed cell death (apoptotic death). When cancer cells die by mitotic death, there is a correlation between cell survival and the number of dicentric and ring chromosomes. Cells that die through apoptotic death have no chromosomal aberrations: radiation-induced damage typically results in DNA fragmentation.[1] Cells that die by apoptosis (e.g., lymphoma cells) have no dose–rate effect. In contrast, cells that die a mitotic death (i.e., most solid tumors, including prostate cancer) possess a dose–rate effect. Thus, radiotherapy for lymphoma requires a lower dose (usually 20–40 Gy), whereas in most solid tumors, the definitive dose is in the range of 70–80 Gy.

The presence of oxygen in solid tumors significantly influences the biological effect of radiation. In the absence of oxygen, radiation-induced cell damage may be repaired. Although hypoxic fractions in solid tumors vary, hypoxia can decrease local control of solid tumors. It is unknown to which degree hypoxia affects radiation efficacy and progression-free survival in patients with prostate cancer.

In prostate cancer radiotherapy, one typically uses small daily fractions of radiation, so-called *conventional fractionation*, which employs 1.8–2.0 Gy daily fractions. The basis of conventional fractionation is that splitting a dose into smaller fractions spares normal tissue due to sublethal damage repair and cellular repopulation, while at the same time increasing tumor damage to dividing cancer cells. Fraction size is an important factor in determining late effects to normal tissues after radiotherapy: Higher fraction size is associated with higher risk for late toxicities to normal tissues. *Hypofractionation*, which employs daily fractions greater than 2 Gy, is an attractive approach in radiotherapy for localized prostate cancer since radiotherapy can be completed within 2–3 weeks, in comparison with conventionally fractionated radiotherapy, which takes 7–8 weeks. This certainly can reduce the economic burden of prostate cancer radiotherapy; however, potential late toxicities to normal tissues (such as the rectum and bladder) with a hypofractionated regimen remain a problem. Further research with prospective randomized trials with 5 or more years of follow-up is necessary to establish the role of hypofractionation in prostate cancer radiotherapy. Although first results with hypofractionation for prostate cancer are promising,[2,3] they are not yet mature enough to support its routine use in the clinic.

Radiation Therapy: External Beam and Brachytherapy

External Beam Radiation Therapy

In the context of radiation oncology, patients with localized prostate cancer have two treatment options: external beam radiotherapy and brachytherapy. The majority of patients receive external beam radiotherapy, while brachytherapy is used for selected patients with localized prostate cancer. External beam radiotherapy is typically delivered using intensity-modulated radiation therapy (IMRT). This is an advanced form of external beam radiotherapy that allows the delivery of high-dose focused radiation to the prostate while sparing normal tissues. Historically, four-field, whole-pelvis radiotherapy was used to a dose of 45 Gy, followed by a boost to the prostate to a total dose of 65–70 Gy. With IMRT, a higher dose can be delivered to the prostate, while normal tissue toxicity is still low. It has been shown that dose escalation is associated with improved freedom from biochemical failure (i.e., prostate-specific antigen [PSA] progression).[4–9] According to the National Comprehensive Cancer Network (NCCN) guidelines, a dose of 75.6–79.0 Gy in conventional 1.8–2.0 Gy fractions is recommended for patients with low-risk prostate cancers, whereas in patients with intermediate- and high-risk prostate cancer, doses between 78 and 80 Gy are recommended.[10]

Daily image guidance is strongly recommended with dose escalation (Figs. 8.1 and 8.2).[11] This can be done using image-guided radiotherapy with daily cone beam computed tomography (CT) scan prior to each fraction of radiotherapy, ultrasound, or implanted fiducials. A new approach is electromagnetic transponder implant tracking, which does not require daily image guidance (Fig. 8.3). Some facilities even use an endorectal balloon to immobilize the prostate; this can reduce the dose to the lateral and posterior rectal wall, although the dose to the anterior wall of the rectum is inevitably high. The balloon is placed prior to each fraction of radiotherapy. At the University of California Davis, 79.2 Gy in 1.8 Gy fractions is typically delivered over a

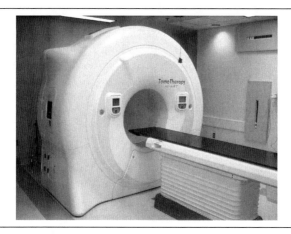

Figure 8.1 TomoTherapy Hi-Art System installed at the University of California, Davis. This system combines integrated computed tomography (CT) imaging with conformal radiation therapy to deliver sophisticated radiation treatments with precision while reducing radiation exposure to surrounding healthy tissue. In this system, a linear accelerator rotates on a ring-gantry. Intensity-modulated radiation therapy treatment is delivered while the couch is translated through the gantry bore in the same way as helical CT imaging is conducted. Photo courtesy of UC Davis Department of Radiation Oncology (See Color plate).

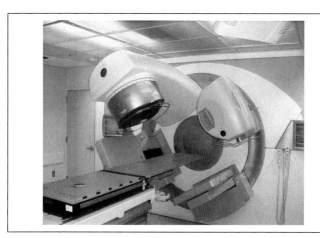

Figure 8.2 Elekta Synergy S installed at the University of California, Davis. Elekta Synergy S is a linear accelerator with 3D image guidance; it allows radiation oncologists to visualize tumor and normal tissue and their movement between fractions. This enables imaging of the patient in the treatment position prior to each fraction of radiation therapy, and delivery of radiation therapy to tumor while sparing normal tissue. Photo courtesy of UC Davis Department of Radiation Oncology (See Color plate).

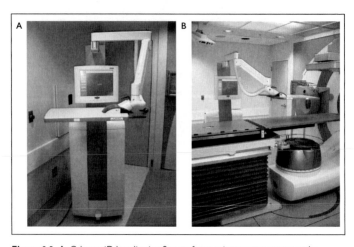

Figure 8.3 A: Calypso 4D Localization System for treating prostate cancer at the University of California, Davis. This technology works like a global positioning system (GPS). It determines the exact position and movement of the prostate during radiation therapy. Three tiny beacon electromagnetic transponders are implanted into the prostate in an outpatient procedure, similar to a biopsy. Each transponder is as small as a grain of rice. The beacon transponders in the prostate communicate with the Calypso 4D Localization System using safe radiofrequency waves. **B:** Calypso 4D Localization System and Elekta Synergy S linear accelerator ready for patient set-up and radiation therapy delivery. Photos courtesy of UC Davis Department of Radiation Oncology (See Color plate).

period of 7.5 weeks with daily image guidance using IMRT with daily CT, or electromagnetic transponder implant tracking.

Brachytherapy

Prostate brachytherapy (as monotherapy) is indicated in patients with low-risk prostate cancer. For patients with intermediate-risk prostate cancer, external beam radiotherapy with IMRT to total dose of 45 Gy, followed by a prostate brachytherapy boost with 4–6 months of neoadjuvant, concurrent, and adjuvant androgen deprivation therapy (ADT), can be considered. Patients with high-risk prostate cancer are generally considered poor candidates for prostate brachytherapy, although with the addition of external beam radiotherapy and ADT, it may still be effective in selected patients (Table 8.1).

A patient with a very large prostate, symptoms of bladder outlet obstruction, or previous transurethral resection of the prostate (TURP) is more difficult to treat with brachytherapy and has an increased risk of side effects. It is important to note that prior TURP is not an absolute contraindication for prostate brachytherapy. If magnetic resonance imaging (MRI) shows a small defect in the prostate, prostate brachytherapy with peripheral seed loading may still be feasible. In patients with a large prostate (>60 cc) and significant obstructive urinary symptoms (high International Prostate Symptom Score [IPSS] score), neoadjuvant ADT should be administered first if brachytherapy is being planned; this can shrink the prostate to an acceptable size for seed implantation. The American

Table 8.1 Absolute and Relative Contraindications for Low-dose-rate (LDR) Prostate Brachytherapy (Seed Implantation) with ^{125}Iodine or ^{103}Palladium

Absolute Contraindications	• Severe obstructive urinary symptoms[A] (International Prostate Symptom [IPS] score ≥16 despite α-blocker therapy)
	• History of urethral stricture
	• Medically poor surgical candidate (unable to undergo general anesthesia)
Relative Contraindications	• Moderate obstructive urinary symptoms (IPS score <15) but patient requiring continuous use of α-blocker therapy[B]
	• Prior history of transurethral resection of the prostate (TURP)[C]
	• Prostate gland >60 cc (unless androgen deprivation therapy is given for 2–3 months for prostate volume reduction[D])

[A] 80–90% of patients after brachytherapy develop grade 1 urinary toxicities such as nocturia, and irritative symptoms with peaks approximately 2 weeks following brachytherapy. For this reason, brachytherapy is not considered in patients who already have severe obstructive urinary symptoms.

[B] α-Blockers such as tamsulosin or terazosin.

[C] Magnetic resonance imaging (MRI) of the prostate should be obtained to evaluate for post-TURP volume defect in the prostate. If the defect is small, LDR brachytherapy with peripheral seed loading may still be feasible.

[D] Transurethral prostate ultrasound should be performed and prostate volume should be measured after androgen deprivation therapy. If the volume is <60 cc, LDR brachytherapy can be reconsidered.

Brachytherapy Society (ABS) recommends monotherapy prescribed doses for ^{125}Iodine and ^{103}Palladium to be 145 Gy and 125 Gy, respectively. For external beam radiotherapy with ^{125}Iodine or ^{103}Palladium boost, the ABS recommends boost doses of 100–110 Gy and 90–100 Gy, respectively[12] (Table 8.2).

Multi-institutional, long-term results of prostate brachytherapy are excellent, with 8-year PSA progression-free survival rates of 93%,[13] and 10-year progression-free survival rates of 87%.[14] A PSA nadir of 0.5 ng/mL or less was particularly associated with durable long-term PSA disease-free survival, and the only controllable factor to impact on long-term outcome was a dose to 90% of the prostate (D90), which is a reflection of implant quality.[13] Figure 8.4 shows a post-treatment pelvic CT scan of a patient who received LDR brachytherapy with ^{125}Iodine seed implantation.

Prophylactic Pelvic Nodal Irradiation

Prophylactic pelvic nodal irradiation can be considered in the treatment of high-risk patients, although at this time there is no strong evidence to support routine pelvic nodal irradiation. The concept of whole-pelvic radiotherapy for patients with high-risk prostate cancer is based on the assumption that these patients can potentially harbor micrometastasis in the pelvic lymph nodes. This concept, however, remains controversial. The Radiation Therapy Oncology

Table 8.2 Clinical Criteria for Low-dose-rate Brachytherapy (Seed Implantation) with ¹²⁵Iodine or ¹⁰³Palladium

Radiation Therapy (RT)	Clinical Criteria[A]
LDR brachytherapy alone	Clinical stage T1–T2a
	Gleason score ≤6, or low volume Gleason 3 + 4[B]
	PSA ≤10
External beam RT combined with LDR brachytherapy[D]	Clinical stage T2b–T2c
	High volume Gleason score 3 + 4[C]
	Gleason score 4 + 3
	PSA >10–≤20

LDR = low dose rate.

[A] Clinical criteria may vary from institution to institution.

[B] ≤50% biopsy cores involved.

[C] >50% biopsy cores involved.

[D] If combined approach is contemplated, external beam RT to the prostate and proximal (1 cm) seminal vesicles to total dose of 45 Gy in 1.8 Gy fractions is delivered first. It is optional to include the entire seminal vesicles. Intensity-modulated radio therapy (IMRT) can be used for external beam RT component.

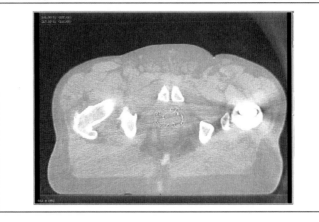

Figure 8.4 Post-treatment pelvic computed tomography (CT) scan of a 67-year-old man with a low-risk prostate cancer status post low-dose-rate (LDR) brachytherapy with ¹²⁵Iodine seed implantation. Note peripheral seed loading in the prostate, and isodose lines: 100% isodose line is in green and 150% isodose line is in blue. A radiation oncologist, urologist, and radiation oncology physicist perform the procedure in an operating room (See Color plate).

Group (RTOG) 9413 clinical trial initially showed improved 4-year progression-free survival with whole-pelvic radiotherapy in patients with estimated risk of lymph node involvement of 15%.[15] Whole-pelvic radiotherapy was associated with a 4-year progression-free survival of 54%, compared with 47% in patients treated with radiotherapy to the prostate alone ($p = 0.022$). However, with a longer follow-up of RTOG 9413, the improvement in progression-free survival with whole-pelvic radiotherapy versus prostate-only radiotherapy was no longer significant.[16]

Although the results of RTOG 9413 are provocative, they are difficult to accept as evidence in support of whole-pelvic radiotherapy, given the lack of understanding of why these results changed with longer follow-up. King and Kapp recently proposed a hypothesis that larger scatter dose to the testes with whole-pelvic radiotherapy compared with prostate-only radiotherapy can have a negative effect on testosterone production, which is proportional to the dose to the testes (or more precisely the Leydig cells). According to this hypothesis, an increase in time to testosterone recovery leads to a delay in biochemical failure, and therefore gives an apparent but temporary advantage for whole-pelvic radiotherapy. The cumulative scatter dose from a course of whole-pelvic radiotherapy (45–50 Gy) followed by prostate boost (25 Gy) is calculated to be within the range of 4.3 to 9.1 Gy.[17]

Radiation Therapy vis a vis Radical Prostatectomy

Kupelian and colleagues retrospectively analyzed the biochemical progression-free survival in 2,991 consecutive patients treated at the Cleveland Clinic Foundation, and at Memorial Sloan Kettering at Mercy Medical Center. The majority of patients had low- and intermediate-risk prostate cancer character-ized by clinical stage T1c and T2a (92% of patients) and Gleason score ≤ 7 (93% of patients). Mean PSA value in this group was 11 ng/mL. The 7-year biochemical relapse-free survival rate for radical prostatectomy, external beam radiotherapy of 72 Gy or more, prostate brachytherapy, and external beam radiotherapy combined with prostate brachytherapy was 76%, 81%, 75%, and 77%, respectively. The biochemical failure rates were similar among different treatment modalities, and the patients' characteristics (stage, PSA, and Gleason score) were fairly equally distributed among the treatment groups.[18] This sug-gests that radiotherapy for low- and intermediate-risk patients is as effective as radical prostatectomy for the same risk groups of patients. However, no adequately powered prospective trials comparing these modalities directly are available.

Radiation Therapy with Androgen Deprivation Therapy

Radiotherapy with ADT is given to patients with intermediate- and high-risk prostate cancer. In patients with intermediate-risk disease, ADT is typically administered for 4–6 months, whereas in high-risk patients, it is administered for 2–3 years or in some cases, even longer. Androgen deprivation therapy is not recommended for patients with low-risk disease. Androgen deprivation therapy consists of a luteinizing-hormone releasing-hormone (LHRH) agonist, such as goserelin and leuprolide, and an androgen receptor blocker, such as flutamide and bicalutamide. With IMRT, ADT is administered 8–12 weeks prior to initiation of radiotherapy. At the University of California Davis, subcutaneous goserelin 10.8 mg is typically prescribed every 3 months, and bicalutamide 50 mg/day orally daily for at least 2 months. Bicalutamide is initiated with the first injection of goserelin. After an initial period of total androgen blockade, LHRH agonist is continued for the rest of ADT.

Radiation Therapy with Short-term Androgen Deprivation Therapy

In patients with intermediate-risk disease, a phase III study from the United States enrolling 206 patients showed that short-term ADT (6 months) with external beam radiotherapy (70 Gy) improves PSA control and overall survival.[19] In this study, Kaplan-Meier estimates of 5-year survival rates were 88% in the combined arm versus 78% in the radiotherapy alone arm. Rates of survival free of salvage ADT at 5 years were 82% in the combined arm versus 57% in the radiotherapy-alone arm.

Another phase III study from Australia enrolling 818 patients confirmed that short-term ADT with external beam radiotherapy (66 Gy) improved the outlook in patients with locally advanced prostate cancer. The study showed that 6-month ADT significantly improved local failure, biochemical failure-free survival, disease-free survival, freedom from salvage treatment, distant failure, and prostate cancer–specific survival compared with no androgen deprivation[20] (Figs. 8.5a and 8.5b).

Radiation Therapy with Long-term Androgen Deprivation Therapy

As previously mentioned, in patients with high-risk prostate cancer, the recommended duration of ADT is 2–3 years with external beam radiotherapy. The landmark trial from the European Organization for Research and Treatment of Cancer (EORTC 22961) phase III study showed that ADT for 3 years with external beam radiotherapy (70 Gy) improved biochemical disease-free survival and overall survival.[21] In this study, which included 415 patients, 5-year disease-free survival was 40% in the radiotherapy-alone arm and 74% in the combined treatment arm ($p = 0.0001$); 5-year overall survival was 62% in the radiotherapy-alone arm and 78% in the combined treatment arm ($p = 0.0002$).

In the RTOG 9202 study, 1,554 patients were randomly assigned to receive external beam radiotherapy (65–70 Gy) with 4 months versus 24 months of ADT. The long-term ADT arm showed significant improvement in all efficacy endpoints except overall survival (OS; 80.0% vs. 78.5% at 5 years, $p = 0.73$), compared with the short-term ADT arm.[22] In a subset of patients who were not part of the original study design, with cancers assigned Gleason scores of 8–10, the long-term ADT arm had significantly better OS (81.0% vs 70.7%, $p = 0.044$).

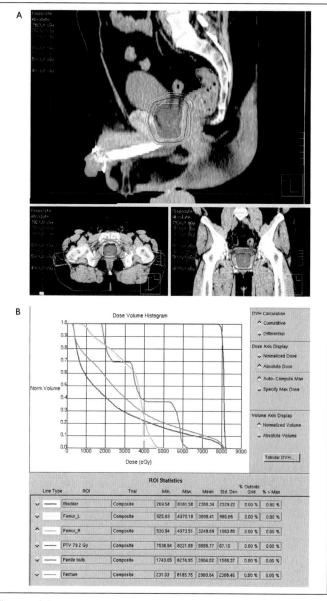

Figure 8.5A,B: Intensity-modulated radiation therapy (IMRT) plan of a 50-year-old man with intermediate-risk prostate cancer. He received 55.8 Gy in 1.8 Gy fractions to the prostate and proximal seminal vesicles, followed by boost to the prostate to a total dose of 79.2 Gy, along with 6 months of androgen deprivation therapy. The red area shows prostate with a treatment margin, the so-called the planning target volume (PTV). Thin lines around the PTV represent isodose distribution. Blue contour shows the bladder and orange contour the rectum (See Color plate).

Although the current approach in radiation oncology is to combine ADT and to escalate the dose of radiotherapy with IMRT to 79–80 Gy, it is important to note that the clinical trials supporting the combination of external beam radiotherapy with ADT all used doses of 70 Gy or less. In contrast, most dose-escalation trials did not use ADT. Therefore, it is unclear whether ADT is really beneficial in the setting of dose escalation. To address this question, the RTOG recently opened a phase III trial of dose-escalated radiotherapy with or without short-term (6 months) ADT for patients with intermediate-risk prostate cancer (RTOG 0815). The primary objective of this clinical trial is to determine whether the addition of short-term ADT to dose-escalated radiotherapy has an overall survival advantage compared to dose-escalated radiotherapy alone (Table 8.3).

More recently, a multicenter, randomized phase III study of ADT plus radiation therapy in patients with locally advanced prostate cancer assessed the effect of radiation on overall survival when added to lifelong AD.[23] In this trial, patients with T3/T4 or T2 disease, with PSA levels of greater than 40 μg/L, or T2 disease with PSA levels of greater than 20 μg/L *and* a Gleason score of 8 or more *and* N0/NX, M0 prostate adenocarcinoma were randomized to life-long ADT (bilateral orchiectomy or LHRH agonist) with or without radiation therapy (65–69 Gy to prostate ± seminal vesicles with or without 45Gy to pelvic nodes). In this study, the addition of radiation to lifelong ADT reduced the risk of death (hazard ratio [HR] 0.77, 95% confidence interval [CI] 0.61–0.98, $p = 0.033$) significantly. Disease-specific survival was also in favor of the combination arm, with a HR of 0.57 (95% CI 0.41–0.81, $p = 0.001$).

Adjuvant and Salvage Radiation Therapy

Although radical prostatectomy is an effective treatment option for patients with localized prostate cancer, postprostatectomy relapse in the prostate bed is possible with biochemical progression as the only sign of relapse. An early single-institution study from Thomas Jefferson University showed that adjuvant radiotherapy for pT3N0 prostate cancer could significantly reduce the risk of PSA failure when compared with radical prostatectomy alone.[24] Recent multi-institutional matched-control analysis of adjuvant and salvage postoperative radiotherapy for pT3–4N0 prostate cancer, which included 449 patients, showed that early adjuvant radiotherapy significantly reduces the risk of long-term biochemical progression compared with salvage radiotherapy.[25] Three prospective randomized clinical trials, EORTC 22911,[26] SWOG 8794,[27] and the German Cancer Society ARO 96–02 trial[28] demonstrated improved biochemical progression-free survival with immediate postoperative radiotherapy to the surgical prostate bed in patients with pathologic T3 disease and positive surgical margins. Table 8.4 gives a brief summary of prospective randomized trials for adjuvant radiation therapy to the prostate bed. Secondary analysis of EORTC 22911 showed that margin status is the most important predictor of biochemical progression-free survival.[29] A long-term follow-up of the SWOG 8794 trial[30] with median follow-up of 12.7 years showed that adjuvant radio-

Table 8.3 Current Approaches in Prostate Cancer Radiation Therapy

Risk groups	Stage	Gleason Score	PSA	Radiation Therapy (RT) [A]	Androgen Deprivation Therapy (ADT)
Low risk	T1–T2a, and	2–6, and	≤10 ng/mL	Prostate only, IMRT, 79.2 Gy in 1.8 Gy fractions, or low-dose-rate (LDR) brachytherapy alone	No
Intermediate risk	T2b–T2c, or	7, or	>10–≤20 ng/mL	Prostate + proximal seminal vesicles (1 cm) to 55.8 Gy, followed by boost to the prostate to a total dose of 79.2 Gy, IMRT[B] in 1.8 Gy fractions. External beam RT with IMRT (45 Gy) followed by LDR brachytherapy is possible in selected patients (refer to brachytherapy in the chapter)	Consider 6 months of ADT[C], especially in patients with high intermediate-risk feature: ≥50% biopsy cores involved
High risk	T3a, or	8–10, or	>20 ng/mL	External beam RT with IMRT to a total dose of 79.2 Gy as for intermediate-risk patients; it is optional to include the entire seminal vesicles. Consider pelvic lymph node RT[D] in patients with Gleason score ≥9 or patients with enlarged pelvic lymph nodes (gross disease)	2–3 years of ADT[C]

[A] Radiotherapy doses may vary slightly from institution to institution; in general, external beam dose escalation (78–80 Gy) is now widely used based on the dose-escalation trials published over the past decade (refer to the text).

[B] If ADT is recommended, ADT is given first for at least 8 weeks prior to RT start. This period of time allows the prostate to shrink, thus reducing rectal dose and potential rectal toxicity from RT.

[C] ADT consists of an androgen receptor blocker (ARB) e.g., bicalutamide, 50 mg PO daily, and an LHRH agonist, e.g., goserelin, 10.8 mg s.q., every 3 months. Treatment with ARB should be started at the same time as treatment with an LHRH agonist. Liver function test should be obtained prior to initiation of ARB therapy. ARB therapy is given for the first 2–4 months of ADT, and then LHRH agonist is continued alone.

[D] Prophylactic pelvic lymph node dose is typically 45 Gy. Higher doses of 50–55 Gy should be considered when lymph nodes are enlarged (gross disease). The proximity of the small bowel loops does not allow further pelvic lymph node dose escalation.

Table 8.4 Summary of Prospective Randomized Trials for Adjuvant Radiation Therapy to the Prostate Bed

Clinical trial and number of patients	Patients characteristics	Arms[A,B]	Outcome[C]
• SWOG 8794[25,27] • 425 patients between 1988–1997	• pT3N0M0 • 87% with Gleason ≤ 7 • 66% with postop PSA <0.2 ng/mL	RT (60–64 Gy) vs. observation	• Median PSA relapse-free survival 10.3 yrs for RT vs. 3.1 yrs for observation (p <0.001) • Median recurrence-free survival 13.8 yrs for RT vs. 9.9 yrs for observation (p = 0.001) • Median metastasis-free survival 12.9 yrs for RT vs. 14.7 yrs for observation (p = 0.016) • Median overall survival 13.3 yrs for RT vs. 15.2 yrs for observation (p = 0.023)
• EORTC 22911[24] • 503 patients between 1992–2001	• pT3N0M0 • Approx. 2/3 of patients with positive margins • 86% with WHO histological grade 2–3 • 70% with postop PSA <0.2 ng/mL	RT (60 Gy) vs. observation	• Biochemical progression-free survival was 74% for RT and 52.6% for observation (p < 0.0001) • Clinical progression-free survival was improved (p = 0.0009), and locoregional failure was lowered with adjuvant RT (p < 0.0001). • No significant difference in overall survival with 5-year median follow-up (p = 0.679)
• ARO 96–02[26] • 388 patients between 1997–2004	• pT3N0M0 • Approx. 2/3 of patients with positive margins • 86% with Gleason ≤7 • 80% with postop PSA <0.1	RT (60 Gy) vs. observation	• Biochemical progression-free survival was 72% for RT and 54% for observation (p = 0.015) • No significant difference in overall survival with 4.4-year median follow-up.

[A] Radiation therapy after prostatectomy began within 4 months in SWOG 8794, a median period of 3 months in EORTC 22911, and 3 months in ARO 96–02.

[B] Currently, the majority of radiation oncologists deliver between 64.8 and 70.2 Gy (1.8 Gy fractions) with IMRT.

[C] Median follow-up was the following: 12.7 yrs in SWOG 8794, 5 yrs in EORTC 22911, and 4.4 yrs in ARO 96–02.

therapy improves metastasis-free survival and overall survival. With adjuvant radiotherapy, median overall survival was improved by 1.7 years.

There are no phase III trials guiding the eligibility for salvage radiotherapy. Hence, salvage radiotherapy is indicated if risk of local disease is high and risk of distant metastases is low. Since there are no imaging modalities that can identify local disease at such low PSA levels, the uncertainty regarding the site of failure still remains. Hayes and Pollack analyzed predictors for lower freedom from biochemical failure (FFBF) and found several factors, which have been related to lower FFBF: Gleason score of more than 7, seminal vesicle invasion, high preradiotherapy PSA (>1.0 ng/mL), short PSA doubling time, negative prostatectomy margins, treatment for a persistently detectable PSA after surgery, palpable prostatic bed mass, and radiotherapy dose of less than 65 Gy.[31] Stephenson and colleagues used multivariable Cox regression analysis to predict the probability of disease progression after salvage radiotherapy in a multi-institutional cohort of 1,540 patients. Nearly half of patients with recurrent prostate cancer after radical prostatectomy have a long-term PSA response to salvage radiotherapy when treatment is administered at the earliest sign of recurrence. Four-year progression-free probability was 52% in patients with preradiotherapy PSA levels of 2 or less versus 19% in patients with preradiotherapy PSA levels of more than 2.0. The highest 4-year progression-free probability of 69% was found in patients with preradiotherapy PSA levels of 2 or less, Gleason score of 7 or less, positive surgical margins, and PSA doubling time of greater than 10 months[32] (Fig. 8.6).

At this time, it is unclear whether postprostatectomy patients with a negative bone scan and an isolated PSA failure have subclinical bony metastases. In such patients, the PSA failure may be driven mostly by subclinical bony metastases; the administration of β-emitting bone-targeted therapy with [153]Samarium could result in a measurable decline in the PSA. A phase I trial of [153]Samarium for treatment of clinically nonmetastatic high-risk prostate cancer was recently reported.[33] In this study, high-risk M0 prostate cancer patients received a month of ADT, followed by [153]Samarium administration, 4 more months of ADT, and radiotherapy (70.2 Gy). The study demonstrated that 2 mCi/kg [153]Samarium with ADT and radiotherapy is safe and feasible. A phase II study to test this treatment is currently under way by the Radiation Therapy Oncology Group (RTOG 0622). The primary objective of this clinical trial is to assess the effectiveness of [153]Samarium administration, as determined by a 30% decline in the PSA within 12 weeks, as compared to baseline.

Toxicities of Radiation Therapy

For external beam radiotherapy, the acute toxicities include urinary frequency, urinary urgency, dysuria, hematuria, soft stools, diarrhea, and proctitis. Potential late side effects include urinary incontinence, urethral stricture, increased frequency of bowel movements, change of stool caliber, rectal ulceration and rectal bleeding, proctitis, and erectile dysfunction.

Zelefsky et al. analyzed the predictors of late toxicities in 743 patients with localized prostate cancer treated with high-dose 3D conformal radiotherapy.

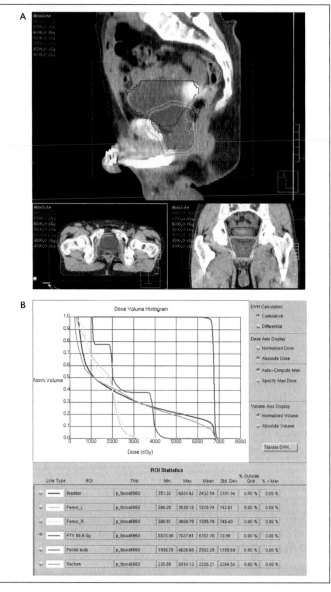

Figure 8.6A,B: Intensity-modulated radiation therapy (IMRT) plan of a 62-year-old man, who achieved undetectable PSA after prostatectomy, and a year later biochemical recurrence with a slowly rising PSA. He received 66.6 Gy in 1.8 Gy fractions to the prostate bed. The red area shows the prostate bed with a treatment margin to account for set-up error and motion. Note that treatment volume includes the vesicourethral anastomosis (right below the bladder), retrovesical space, and bladder neck—these are the most common locations of relapse in the prostate bed after radical prostatectomy.[37] Thin lines around the PTV show isodose distribution (See Color plate).

The 5-year actuarial likelihood of the development of grade 2 and 3 late gastrointestinal toxicities was 11% and 0.75%, respectively. A multivariate analysis identified doses 75.6 Gy or more ($p < 0.001$), history of diabetes mellitus ($P = 0.01$), and the presence of acute gastrointestinal symptoms during treatment ($P = 0.02$) as independent predictors of grade 2 or higher late gastrointestinal toxicity. The 5-year actuarial likelihood of the development of grade 2 and 3 late genitourinary toxicities was 10% and 3%, respectively. Doses of 75.6 Gy or more ($P = 0.008$) and acute genitourinary symptoms ($p <0.001$) were independent predictors of grade 2 or higher late genitourinary toxicity. Overall, the incidence of severe late complications after high-dose 3D conformal radiotherapy was low.[34] Intensity-modulated radiation therapy additionally reduced the incidence of acute and late rectal toxicities compared with 3D conformal radiotherapy, although acute and late urinary toxicities were not significantly different. In 561 patients treated with IMRT and dose escalation (81 Gy), the 8-year actuarial likelihood of grade 2 rectal bleeding was 1.6%. Only 0.1% of patients experienced grade 3 rectal toxicity requiring either one or more transfusions or a laser cauterization procedure. No grade 4 rectal complications have been observed. The 8-year likelihood of late grade 2 and 3 (urethral strictures) urinary toxicities was 9% and 3%, respectively.[6]

For low-dose-rate brachytherapy, the acute side effects include perineal pain and swelling, hematuria, dysuria, urinary frequency and urgency, nocturia, obstructive urinary symptoms, and passing of the implanted seeds. Potential late side effects include seed migration to the lungs, urinary incontinence, urinary retention, rectal ulceration and bleeding, and erectile dysfunction. Obstructive urinary symptoms can be managed with α-blockers, such as tamsulosin and terazosin. Rectal symptoms may require stool softeners to avoid constipation and cortisone suppositories. Invasive procedures, such as laser coagulation, should be avoided due to risk of fistula formation.

The strongest predictor of sexual function after external beam radiotherapy was sexual function prior to treatment. A decrease in sexual function is seen in the first 24 months after external beam radiotherapy, and sexual function is stabilized 2 years after treatment completion. This indicates that sexual function does not have a continuous decline after external beam radiotherapy.[35]

Long-term Outcomes

As discussed earlier, the long-term outcomes of radiotherapy for prostate cancer are comparable to those of radical prostatectomy. Since many high-risk patients will have a positive margin or pathologic T3 disease requiring adjuvant radiotherapy to the prostate fossa, definitive external beam radiotherapy with long-term ADT is being increasingly used for these patients. Although surgery and radiotherapy are main treatment modalities, the question is whether endocrine therapy alone can offer an outcome comparable to that of radiotherapy. To answer this question, the Scandinavian Prostate Cancer Group and Swedish Association for Urological Oncology did a phase III randomized trial including 875 patients with locally advanced prostate cancer (T3 disease in 78% of patients). The patients were randomized between endocrine treatment alone (3 months of total androgen blockade followed by continuous endocrine therapy using flutamide), and the same endocrine therapy combined with radiotherapy (70 Gy). Cumulative incidence at 10 years for prostate cancer–specific mortality and overall mortality was 23.9% and 39.4%, respectively, in the endocrine therapy alone group, and 11.9% and 29.6%, respectively, in the endocrine therapy plus radiotherapy group. Cumulative incidence at 10 years for PSA recurrence was 74.7% in the endocrine therapy alone group versus 25.9% in the endocrine therapy plus radiotherapy group ($p < 0.0001$). The study showed that, in patients with locally advanced prostate cancer, addition of radiotherapy to endocrine therapy improves prostate cancer–specific mortality and overall mortality, and decreases PSA recurrence rate.[36]

Postradiation Follow-up Strategies

For patients initially treated with a curative intent, a serum PSA level should be measured every 6 months for the first 5 years and then checked annually. Digital rectal exam is recommended annually. Patients treated with ADT are at risk for developing osteoporosis. A baseline bone density test should be obtained prior to initiation of ADT. Daily supplementation with calcium (500 mg) and vitamin D (400 IU) is also recommended. Patients who are osteoporotic should be considered for bisphosphonate therapy.

According to the 2006 RTOG/ASTRO/Phoenix consensus definition, a rise of PSA by 2 ng/mL or more above the nadir PSA (defined as the lowest PSA achieved) is currently the standard definition for biochemical failure after external beam radiotherapy with or without ADT.[37] The ASTRO/RTOG consensus also recommended that the date of failure be determined "at call" (not backdated).

For patients with biochemical failure after external beam radiotherapy or brachytherapy, treatment options are observation (if PSA doubling time is not short), initiation of ADT, salvage radical prostatectomy, and cryotherapy. Agarwal and colleagues[38] analyzed treatment failure after primary and salvage radiotherapy for prostate cancer. Using a national disease registry, the Cancer of the Prostate Strategic Urological Research Endeavor (CaPSURE) database, 5,277 men with prostate cancer who initially underwent radical prostatectomy or external beam radiotherapy were identified. Disease recurrence developed in 30% of patients who were treated for prostate cancer, and ADT was the most common salvage therapy used. Salvage radical prostatectomy was used only in 0.9% of patients who failed external beam radiotherapy. The mean time between primary treatment and recurrence was 34 months in radical prostatectomy group, and 38 months in external beam radiotherapy group. Patients who failed salvage therapy had worse overall survival, and no survival benefit was seen for any particular combination of primary and salvage therapy. Lee and colleagues at the University of California, San Francisco retrospectively analyzed 21 patients who underwent salvage high-dose-rate brachytherapy for locally recurrent prostate cancer following external beam radiotherapy. The 2-year estimate of biochemical control after recurrence was 89%. Three patients developed grade 3 genitourinary toxicity. The study showed that salvage high-dose-rate brachytherapy is feasible and effective.[39]

References

1. Hall EJ, Giaccia AJ. *Radiobiology for the Radiobiologist,* 6th ed. Philadelphia: Lippincott Williams & Wilkins, 2006.

2. Miles EF, Lee WR. Hypofractionation for prostate cancer: A critical review. *Semin Radiat Oncol* 2008;18(1):41–47.

3. Ritter M. Rationale, conduct, and outcome using hypofractionated radiotherapy in prostate cancer. *Semin Radiat Oncol* 2008;18(4):249–256.

4. Pollack A, Zagars GK, Starkschall G, et al. Prostate cancer radiation dose response: Results of the M. D. Anderson phase III randomized trial. *Int J Radiat Oncol Biol Phys* 2002;53(5):1097–1105.

5. Hanks GE, Hanlon AL, Epstein B, Horwitz EM. Dose response in prostate cancer with 8–12 years' follow-up. *Int J Radiat Oncol Biol Phys* 2002;54(2):427–435.

6. Zelefsky MJ, Chan H, Hunt M, et al. Long-term outcome of high dose intensity modulated radiation therapy for patients with clinically localized prostate cancer. *J Urol* 2006;176:1415–1419.

7. Zietman AL, DeSilvio ML, Slater JD, et al. Comparison of conventional-dose vs high-dose conformal radiation therapy in clinically localized adenocarcinoma of the prostate: A randomized controlled trial. *JAMA* 2005;294(10):1233–1239.

8. Peeters ST, Heemsbergen WD, Koper PC, et al. Dose-response in radiotherapy for localized prostate cancer: Results of the Dutch multicenter randomized phase III trial comparing 68 Gy of radiotherapy with 78 Gy. *J Clin Oncol* 2006;24(13):1990–1996.

9. Dearnaley DP, Sydes MR, Graham JD, et al. Escalated-dose versus standard-dose conformal radiotherapy in prostate cancer: first results from the MRC RT01 randomised controlled trial. *Lancet Oncol* 2007;8(6):475–487.

10. National Comprehensive Cancer Network Clinical Practice Guidelines in Oncology, Prostate Cancer. Accessed May 31, 2010 at http://www.nccn.org.

11. Valicenti RK, Lin A. Prostate cancer: Overview and treatment guidelines for image-guided radiation therapy. In: Valicenti RK, Dicker AP and Jaffray DA, eds. *Image-guided radiation therapy of prostate cancer.* New York: Informa Healthcare, 2008: 1–8.

12. Rivard MJ, Butler WM, Devlin PM, et al. American Brachytherapy Society recommends no change for prostate permanent implant dose prescriptions using iodine-125 or palladium-103. *Brachytherapy* 2007;6(1):34–37.

13. Zelefsky MJ, Kuban DA, Levy LB, et al. Multi-institutional analysis of long-term outcome for stages T1–T2 prostate cancer treated with permanent seed implantation. *Int J Radiat Oncol Biol Phys* 2007;67(2):327–333.

14. Grimm PD, Blasko JC, Sylvester JE, et al. 10-year biochemical (prostate-specific antigen) control of prostate cancer with (125)I brachytherapy. *Int J Radiat Oncol Biol Phys* 2001;51(1):31–40.

15. Roach M 3rd, DeSilvio M, Lawton C, et al. Phase III trial comparing whole-pelvic versus prostate-only radiotherapy and neoadjuvant versus adjuvant combined androgen suppression: Radiation Therapy Oncology Group 9413. *J Clin Oncol* 2003;21(10):1904–1911.

16. Lawton CA, DeSilvio M, Roach M 3rd, et al. An update of the phase III trial comparing whole pelvic to prostate only radiotherapy and neoadjuvant to adjuvant total androgen suppression: Updated analysis of RTOG 94–13, with emphasis on unexpected hormone/radiation interactions. *Int J Radiat Oncol Biol Phys* 2007;69(3):646–655.

17. King CR, Kapp DS. To treat pelvic nodes or not: Could the greater testicular scatter dose from whole pelvic fields confound results of prostate cancer trials? *J Clin Oncol* 2009;27(36):6076–6078.

18. Kupelian PA, Potters L, Khuntia D, et al. Radical prostatectomy, external beam radiotherapy <72 Gy, external beam radiotherapy ≥ 72 Gy, permanent seed implantation, or combined seeds/external beam radiotherapy for stage T1–T2 prostate cancer. *Int J Radiat Oncol Biol Phys* 2004;58(1):25–33.

19. D'Amico AV, Manola J, Loffredo M, et al. 6-month androgen suppression plus radiation therapy vs radiation therapy alone for patients with clinically localized prostate cancer: A randomized controlled trial. *JAMA* 2004;292(7):821–827.

20. Denham JW, Steigler A, Lamb DS, et al. Short-term androgen deprivation and radiotherapy for locally advanced prostate cancer: Results from the Trans-Tasman Radiation Oncology Group 96.01 randomised controlled trial. *Lancet Oncol* 2005;6(11):841–850.

21. Bolla M, Collette L, Blank L, et al. Long-term results with immediate androgen suppression and external irradiation in patients with locally advanced prostate cancer (an EORTC study): A phase III randomised trial. *Lancet* 2002;360:103–106.

22. Hanks GE, Pajak TF, Porter A, et al. Phase III trial of long-term adjuvant androgen deprivation after neoadjuvant hormonal cytoreduction and radiotherapy in locally advanced carcinoma of the prostate: The Radiation Therapy Oncology Group Protocol 92–02. *J Clin Oncol* 2003;21(21):3972–3978.

23. Warde PR, Mason MD, Sydes MR, et al. Intergroup randomized phase III study of androgen deprivation therapy (ADT) plus radiation therapy (RT) in locally advanced prostate cancer (CaP) (NCIC-CTG, SWOG, MRC-UK, INT: T94–0110; NCT00002633). *J Clin Oncol* 2009;28:7s (Suppl; abstr. CRA4504).

24. Valicenti RK, Gomella LG, Ismail M, et al. The efficacy of early adjuvant radiation therapy for pT3N0 prostate cancer: A matched-pair analysis. *Int J Radiat Oncol Biol Phys* 1999;45:53–58.

25. Trabulsi EJ, Valicenti RK, Hanlon AL, et al. A multi-institutional matched-control analysis of adjuvant and salvage postoperative radiation therapy for pT3–4N0 prostate cancer. *Urology* 2008;72:1298–1302.

26. Bolla M, van Poppel H, Collette L, et al. Postoperative radiotherapy after radical prostatectomy: A randomised controlled trial (EORTC trial 22911). *Lancet* 2005;366:572–578.

27. Thompson IM Jr., Tangen CM, Paradelo J, et al. Adjuvant radiotherapy for pathologically advanced prostate cancer: A randomized clinical trial. *JAMA* 2006;296:2329–2335.

28. Wiegel T, Bottke D, Steiner U, et al. Phase III postoperative adjuvant radiotherapy after radical prostatectomy compared with radical prostatectomy alone in pT3 prostate cancer with postoperative undetectable prostate-specific antigen: ARO 96–02/AUO AP 09/95. *J Clin Oncol* 2009;27:2924–2930.

29. Van der Kwast TH, Bolla M, Van Poppel H, et al. Identification of patients with prostate cancer who benefit from immediate postoperative radiotherapy: EORTC 22911. *J Clin Oncol*. 2007; 25(27): 4178–86.

30. Thompson IM, Tangen CM, Paradelo J, et al. Adjuvant radiotherapy for pathological T3N0M0 prostate cancer significantly reduces risk of metastases and improves survival: Long-term followup of a randomized clinical trial. *J Urol* 2009;181:956–962.

31. Hayes SB, Pollack A. Parameters for treatment decisions for salvage radiation therapy. *J Clin Oncol* 2005;23(32):8204–8211.

32. Stephenson AJ, Scardino PT, Kattan MW, et al. Predicting the outcome of salvage radiation therapy for recurrent prostate cancer after radical prostatectomy. *J Clin Oncol* 2007;25(15):2035–2041.

33. Valicenti RK, Trabulsi E, Intenzo C, et al. A phase I trial of samarium-153-lexidronam complex for treatment of clinically nonmetastatic high-risk prostate cancer: First report of a completed study. *Int J Radiat Oncol Biol Phys* (in press).

34. Zelefsky MJ, Cowen D, Fuks Z, et al. Long-term tolerance of high dose three-dimensional conformal radiotherapy in patients with localized prostate carcinoma. *Cancer* 1999;85(11):2460–2468.

35. Siglin J, Kubicek GJ, Leiby B, Valicenti RK. Time of decline in sexual function after external beam radiotherapy for prostate cancer. *Int J Radiat Oncol Biol Phys* 2010;76(1):31–35.

36. Widmark A, Klepp O, Solberg A, et al. Endocrine treatment, with or without radiotherapy, in locally advanced prostate cancer (SPCG-7/SFUO-3): An open randomised phase III trial. *Lancet* 2009;373:301–308.

37. Roach M 3rd, Hanks G, Thames H Jr., et al. Defining biochemical failure following radiotherapy with or without hormonal therapy in men with clinically localized prostate cancer: Recommendations of the RTOG-ASTRO Phoenix Consensus Conference. *Int J Radiat Oncol Biol Phys* 2006;65(4):965–974.

38. Agarwal PK, Sadetsky N, Konety BR, et al. Cancer of the Prostate Strategic Urological Research Endeavor (CaPSURE). Treatment failure after primary and salvage therapy for prostate cancer: likelihood, patterns of care, and outcomes. *Cancer* 2008;112(2):307–314.

39. Lee B, Shinohara K, Weinberg V, et al. Feasibility of high-dose-rate brachytherapy salvage for local prostate cancer recurrence after radiotherapy: The University of California-San Francisco experience. *Int J Radiat Oncol Biol Phys* 2007;67(4):1106–1112.

Chapter 9

Active Surveillance for Localized Prostate Cancer

Brian Hu and Theresa Koppie

Although surgery and radiation therapy have been utilized in treating prostate cancer since the early 1900s, active surveillance has recently emerged as an important modality for early-stage disease. Active surveillance is a method of managing low-risk prostate cancer that postpones treatment until evidence of aggressive disease. Enthusiasm for active surveillance as a management strategy stems from growing concerns of prostate cancer overtreatment. With the wide use of prostate-specific antigen (PSA) screening, more detected prostate cancers will be deemed clinically "insignificant"; that is, they will have little or no impact on patient survival. Active surveillance can save some of these patients the treatment-related morbidities and psychosocial issues associated with curative therapy.

Early descriptions of nonintervention for prostate cancer took a passive approach. With *watchful waiting*, physicians and patients would wait for the manifestation of symptoms of local or metastatic disease. Interval evaluation of the cancer was not performed, and any opportunity for cure was lost. Intervention while on watchful waiting was reserved for patients with urinary obstruction from locally advanced disease or for those with symptomatic metastases.

The passive approach of watchful waiting has been replaced by a strategy of *active surveillance*. With active surveillance, patients with low-risk prostate cancer are closely monitored, with the goal of identifying and treating more aggressive disease, should it develop. Those who demonstrate progression to more aggressive disease go on to definitive therapy with a curative intent. Active surveillance aims to identify that group of patients with clinically insignificant prostate cancer and save them from treatment-related complications, while selecting out those who are destined to progress and offering them treatment within the window of cure.

Rationale

As noted in Chapter 1, prostate cancer is prevalent, with as many as 70% of men at the age of 80 demonstrating histologic evidence of disease at autopsy.[1] Widespread PSA testing has led to a profound stage migration, with 50%–60%

of newly diagnosed prostate cancers falling into the favorable-risk category.[2] These cancers have a low risk of metastasis and are less likely to impact a patient's overall survival. With this trend, a significant gap now exists between the lifetime risk of being diagnosed with prostate cancer (16%) and the risk of death from the disease (3%).[3]

The increased detection of insignificant prostate cancers, estimated as high as 54%, combined with the tendency toward intervention in the United States, has resulted in considerable prostate cancer overtreatment.[4,5] The survival benefit from curative therapy in favorable risk patients can take years and often decades to be realized, which gives ample opportunity for a patient to succumb to competing comorbidities. Because of this, studies have shown only a small survival benefit when examining outcomes after definitive therapy. For example, the Swedish Randomized Trial showed an absolute risk reduction of only 5% at 10 years among men undergoing radical prostatectomy when compared to those on watchful waiting.[6] Even more striking are the data from the European Randomized Study of Screening for Prostate Cancer. This study demonstrated that in a PSA-screened population, 48 men would need to undergo curative therapy in order to avoid one prostate cancer death.[7] Greater utilization of active surveillance, which helps in further risk stratification, will help minimize the overtreatment of prostate cancer.

In order to know which groups of patients warrant treatment, knowledge of the untreated natural history of localized prostate cancer is important. Albertsen et al. reported that patients with low Gleason-grade cancers had no significant difference in their survival at 15 years from diagnosis compared with the general population.[8] A study by Johansson et al. had similar findings up to 15 years; however, there was a decrease in cancer-specific survival from 89% to 72% in those followed from 15 to 20 years.[9] This study suggested that observation may not be the ideal strategy for those with a long life expectancy. A follow-up analysis by Albertsen et al. examined survival based on a competing risk analysis. These investigators found that the rate of death from low-risk prostate cancer was only 6 per 1,000 person-years at 20 years of follow-up.[10] Those with high-grade cancers, on the other hand, were found to have a much higher rate of cancer-specific death (121 per 1,000 person-years). It is important to note that these studies were performed in the pre-PSA era and may overestimate the risk of prostate cancer death that would be experienced by contemporary patients. These observational studies have shown that patients with low-grade cancers have very low rates of cancer-specific death up to 20 years of follow-up and that these patients are more likely to die of competing causes. However, those with more aggressive cancers are at high risk of death from prostate cancer and benefit from early identification.

Benefits and Risks

Surgery, brachytherapy, external beam radiotherapy, cryotherapy, focal ablative procedures, and primary androgen deprivation are all subject to treatment-related morbidities, with some men experiencing life-long changes to their quality of life. Sanda et al. examined the health-related quality-of-life changes associated with treatments for prostate cancer and found that each treatment produced unique decrements in urinary, sexual, bowel, and hormonal function. Surgery was associated with adverse effects on sexual function and continence, whereas radiation therapy had more adverse gastrointestinal effects. In addition, those who received hormone therapy experienced worse outcomes across multiple quality-of-life domains.[11] The primary benefit of active surveillance is that patients can avoid or delay such treatment-related morbidity.

Active surveillance may also reduce health care costs. In the United States, the cost of prostate cancer treatment is estimated to range from $1.72 billion to $4.75 billion annually.[12] Managing patients with active surveillance rather than immediate radical prostatectomy can potentially decrease prostate cancer treatment costs by 43% to 79% over 15 years.[13]

Some patients on active surveillance will experience progression to more aggressive disease, which is obviously associated with risks. Deferring prostate cancer treatment can result in disease that requires more aggressive and potentially more morbid treatments, such as adjuvant radiation or androgen deprivation therapy. In addition, a patient may be less fit to undergo therapy given the worsening of medical comorbidities with time. Finally, there is the risk that the prostate cancer will move out of the curable range. Fortunately, short- and intermediate-term data for patients on active surveillance suggest that the risk of clinically significant progression is quite low. The reported risk of metastasis at 2–8 years is less than 1%.[14] Furthermore, a delay in surgery of up to 2 years appears to have no impact on pathologic findings at the time of radical prostatectomy (Table 9.1).[15]

There is also a potential psychological impact to untreated prostate cancer. Litwin et al. reported worse mental health profiles among American men on observation compared to those who underwent a radical prostatectomy.[16] This phenomenon may be cultural, as studies evaluating the psychological impact of active surveillance outside of the United States show no psychological detriment to deferring prostate cancer treatment.[17,18]

Table 9.1 Benefits and Risks of Active Surveillance	
Benefits	Delay or avoidance of treatment-related complications
	Decreased rates of overtreatment
	Lower health care costs
Risks	Missed opportunity for cure
	Potentially more adjuvant therapy needed when treating disease progression
	Possible psychological impact of an untreated cancer
	Need for repeat prostate biopsies

Patient Selection

Currently, there are no standard patient selection criteria for active surveillance. Early studies by Epstein et al. from Johns Hopkins evaluated patients who had a radical prostatectomy for T1c disease and defined those with "insignificant" prostate cancer to have a Gleason grade of 6 or less and a total tumor volume of less than 0.2 cm^3.[19] These authors later determined that a pretreatment PSA density of less than 0.15 ng/mL, pretreatment clinical stage of T2 or lower, and the absence of Gleason 4 or 5 on prostate biopsy to be predictive of insignificant prostate cancer upon subsequent radical prostatectomy.[20] Since then, studies have used a variety of selection criteria for active surveillance protocols. Important considerations include patient age, life expectancy, competing comorbidities, clinical stage, PSA, PSA kinetics, biopsy Gleason grade, and tumor volume (Table 9.2).

At the University of California, Davis, our group recommends that patient selection criteria include Gleason score of 6 or less (no pattern 4 or 5), PSA of 10 or less, clinical stage T1–T2a, stable PSA kinetics, less than 33% cores positive, with no core more than 50% positive. We also recommend that a confirmatory biopsy be performed within 6 months of initial biopsy.

Prior to committing to an active surveillance protocol, patients who elect observation can be further evaluated with a repeat prostate biopsy to help correct for biopsy sampling error. A retrospective study by Suardi et al. examined the rate of tumor undergrading using various pretreatment active surveillance criteria from their radical prostatectomy database. The study found a misclassification rate of 14%–27% when defined as upgrading or upstaging to Gleason grade 8 or more, extracapsular extension, seminal vesicle invasion, or lymph node invasion in prostatectomy specimens.[21] Berglund et al. examined the risk of prostate cancer understaging in patients meeting selection criteria for active surveillance by reviewing pathologic findings of repeat prostate biopsies within 3 months of initial biopsy. An increased grade or stage was identified in 27% of patients on repeat biopsy.[22]

Follow-up

Currently, no clear consensus exists as to the optimal strategy for surveillance. We recommend that patients be followed by patient history, digital rectal examination, and PSA at 3- to 6-month intervals. Prostate biopsies are performed at 1- to 2-year intervals. Progression of disease and need for primary therapy is typically defined as worsening grade of cancer on biopsy, increased volume of cancer on biopsy or imaging, more concerning examination, or worsening PSA kinetics. To date, there has not been a validated marker that defines progression for patients on active surveillance. Finding the exact threshold to determine the need for definitive therapy must be individualized to the patient's clinical parameters and overall health (Table 9.3).

Table 9.2 Summary of Active Surveillance Studies

Ref. No.	Eligibility	Mean age	Follow-up (months)	Number of patients	Progression	Outcomes after treatment	OS	CSS
Retrospective								
23	GS≤7, PSA <15ng/dL, cT1c–T2	70	41	27	29%	31% positive margin after RP	89%	100%
24	T1c–T2, PSA <10 ng/mL, PSAD <0.2 ng/mL/cm³, GS≤6, ≤2 biopsy cores positive	66	47	182	32%		90%	99%
14	age ≤75 years PSA≤10 ng/dL, cT1–T2a, GS≤6, ≤3 positive cores	64	29	262	16%	9% BCR after RP		100%
Prospective (Nonrandomized)								
25	cT1c–T2a, PSAD 0.15 ng/mL/cm³, GS≤6 (no 4 or 5), ≤2 cores positive, no >50% of a single core positive	66	41	407	25%	20% of RP with in curable pathology*	98%	100%
26	PSA ≤15 ng/dL, cT1–T2a, GS <7 (3 + 4) <50% of samples positive, <10 mm of any core	67	22	326	20%	5% BCR after RP	98%	100%
27	PSA <10 ng/mL GS ≤6 (no 4 or 5) <33% of biopsy cores, cT1–T2a	63	43	321	37%	No metastatic disease, BCR after RP 1.3%	100%	100%
28	GS ≤6 or 7, PSA ≤10–15 ng/dL 1 core, life expectancy >10 yrs	70	82	450	30%	50% BCR after RP	82%	10 yr 97%

*pT2 organ confined if Gleason sum was 7 or greater (4 + 3) and/or the surgical margins were positive any grade, stage pT3aN0 if Gleason sum was 7 or greater and/or surgical margins were positive, any stage higher than pT3a regardless of grade or margin status or any N stage

OS, overall survival; CSS, cancer-specific survival; PSAD, PSA density; GS, Gleason score; BCR, biochemical recurrence; RP, radical prostatectomy

Table 9.3 Recommendations for Eligibility and Follow-up	
Eligibility	Gleason ≤6 (no pattern 4 or 5), PSA ≤10, cT1–T2a, stable PSA kinetics, <33% cores positive, no core >50% positive
	Confirmatory biopsy within 6 months of initial biopsy
Follow-up	Biopsy every 1–2 years as indicated by clinical parameters
	DRE and PSA every 3–6 months

Outcomes

There are several published studies on active surveillance[14,23–28] (see Table 9.2). These studies provide promising data for patients on various active surveillance protocols. The data, however, are limited by length of follow-up. In all of the literature to date, there are over 2,000 patients with a median follow-up ranging from 2 to 7 years. Although all studies have different inclusion criteria, there are some common outcomes. Approximately one out of three patients will go on to delayed treatment. The majority of these are due to disease progression by clinical criteria, although some were driven by patient preference. The criteria that drive patients and physicians toward definitive therapy are usually PSA and/or PSA kinetics.[29,30] Studies have shown overall survival rates between 82% and 100%. Most patients died of competing causes, with encouraging cancer-specific survival rates of between 97% and 100%.

Future of Active Surveillance

Ongoing randomized control trials compare active surveillance to initial definitive treatment. The Standard Treatment Against Restricted Treatment (START) trial is led by the National Cancer Institute of Canada. Patients in this trial are randomly assigned to immediate treatment (radical prostatectomy, brachytherapy, or external beam radiation) or active surveillance, with the primary endpoint of disease-specific survival. The Prostate Testing for Cancer and Treatment (PROTECT) trial is currently accruing patients in the United Kingdom. Patients on this trial are being randomly assigned to active surveillance, radical prostatectomy, or radiation therapy.

Conclusion

Although widespread PSA screening has decreased prostate cancer mortality, it has also led to a large number of patients being overtreated. Active surveillance is a method of managing localized, low-risk prostate cancer with postponement of immediate treatment until there is evidence of progression to more aggressive disease. This method can identify more aggressive prostate cancer for definitive local therapy while saving patients with clinically insignificant cancers from treatment-related complications. Studies with intermediate-length follow-up (<10 years) demonstrate it to be a safe treatment option with a very low risk of cancer-specific mortality.

References

1. Rullis I, Shaeffer JA, Lilien OM. Incidence of prostatic carcinoma in the elderly. *Urology* 1975;6:295–297.

2. Cooperberg MR, Moul JW, Carroll PR. The changing face of prostate cancer. *J Clin Oncol* 2005;23(32):8146–8151.

3. Jemal A, Tiwari RC, Murray T, et al. Cancer statistics, 2004. *CA Cancer J Clin* 2004;54:8–29.

4. Schröder FH. Screening for prostate cancer (PC)—an update on recent findings of the European Randomized Study of Screening for Prostate Cancer (ERSPC). *Urol Oncol* 2008;26(5):533–541.

5. Cooperberg MR, Broering JM, Carroll PR. Time trends and local variation in primary treatment of localized prostate cancer. *J Clin Oncol* 2010;28(7):1117–1123.

6. Bill-Axelson A, Holmberg L, Ruutu M, et al. Radical prostatectomy versus watchful waiting in early prostate cancer. *N Engl J Med* 2005;352(19):1977–1984.

7. Schröder FH, Hugosson J, Roobol MJ, et al., for ERSPC Investigators. Screening and prostate-cancer mortality in a randomized European study. *N Engl J Med* 2009;360(13):1320–1328.

8. Albertsen PC, Fryback DG, Storer BE, et al. Long-term survival among men with conservatively treated localized prostate cancer. *JAMA* 1995;274(8):626–631.

9. Johansson JE, Andrén O, Andersson SO, et al. Natural history of early, localized prostate cancer. *JAMA* 2004;291(22):2713–9.

10. Albertsen PC, Hanley JA, Fine J. 20-year outcomes following conservative management of clinically localized prostate cancer. *JAMA* 2005;293(17):2095–2101.

11. Sanda MG, Dunn RL, Michalski J, et al. Quality of life and satisfaction with outcome among prostate-cancer survivors. *N Engl J Med* 2008;358(12):1250–1261.

12. Saigal CS, Litwin MS. The economic costs of early stage prostate cancer. *Pharmacoeconomics* 2002;20(13):869–878.

13. Corcoran AT, Peele PB, Benoit RM. Cost comparison between watchful waiting with active surveillance and active treatment of clinically localized prostate cancer. *Urology* 2010 Apr 8 (Epub ahead of print).

14. Eggener SE, Mueller A, Berglund RK, et al. A multi-institutional evaluation of active surveillance for low risk prostate cancer. *J Urol* 2009;181(4):1635–1641.

15. Warlick C, Trock BJ, Landis P, et al. Delayed versus immediate surgical intervention and prostate cancer outcome. *J Natl Cancer Inst* 2006;98(5):355–357.

16. Litwin MS, Lubeck DP, Spitalny GM, et al. Mental health in men treated for early stage prostate carcinoma: a posttreatment, longitudinal quality of life analysis from the Cancer of the Prostate Strategic Urologic Research Endeavor. *Cancer* 2002;95(1):54–60.

17. Steineck G, Helgesen F, Adolfsson J, et al. Quality of life after radical prostatectomy or watchful waiting. *N Engl J Med* 2002;347(11):790–796.

18. Burnet KL, Parker C, Dearnaley D, et al. Does active surveillance for men with localized prostate cancer carry psychological morbidity? *BJU Int* 2007;100(3):540–543.

19. Epstein JI, Walsh PC, Carmichael M, Brendler CB. Pathologic and clinical findings to predict tumor extent of nonpalpable (stage T1c) prostate cancer. *JAMA* 1994;271(5):368–374.

20. Bastian PJ, Mangold LA, Epstein JI, Partin AW. Characteristics of insignificant clinical T1c prostate tumors. A contemporary analysis. *Cancer* 2004;101(9):2001–2005.

21. Suardi N, Capitanio U, Chun FK, et al. Currently used criteria for active surveillance in men with low-risk prostate cancer: an analysis of pathologic features. *Cancer* 2008;113(8):2068–2072.

22. Berglund RK, Masterson TA, Vora KC, et al. Pathological upgrading and up staging with immediate repeat biopsy in patients eligible for active surveillance. *J Urol* 2008;180(5):1964–1967.

23. Roemeling S, Roobol MJ, de Vries SH, et al. Active surveillance for prostate cancers detected in three subsequent rounds of a screening trial: characteristics, PSA doubling times, and outcome. *Eur Urol* 2007;51(5):1244–1245.

24. van den Bergh RC, Roemeling S, Roobol MJ, et al. Outcomes of men with screen-detected prostate cancer eligible for active surveillance who were managed expectantly. *Eur Urol* 2009;55(1):1–8

25. Carter HB, Kettermann A, Warlick C, et al. Expectant management of prostate cancer with curative intent: an update of the Johns Hopkins experience. *J Urol* 2007;178(6):2359–2364.

26. van As NJ, Parker CC. Active surveillance with selective radical treatment for localized prostate cancer. *Cancer J* 2007;13(5):289–294.

27. Dall'Era MA, Konety BR, Cowan JE, et al. Active surveillance for the management of prostate cancer in a contemporary cohort. *Cancer* 2008;112(12):2664–2670.

28. Klotz L, Zhang L, Lam A, et al. Clinical results of long-term follow-up of a large, active surveillance cohort with localized prostate cancer. *J Clin Oncol* 2010;28(1):126–131.

29. Koppie TM, Grossfeld GD, Miller D, et al. Patterns of treatment of patients with prostate cancer initially managed with surveillance: results from The CaPSURE database. Cancer of the Prostate Strategic Urological Research Endeavor. *J Urol* 2000;164(1):81–88.

30. Meng MV, Elkin EP, Harlan SR, et al. Predictors of treatment after initial surveillance in men with prostate cancer: results from CaPSURE. *J Urol* 2003;170(6 Pt 1): 2279–2283.

Chapter 10

Advanced or Metastatic Prostate Cancer: Treatment Strategies for Hormone-naïve Disease

Primo N. Lara, Jr.

Metastatic prostate cancer is an incurable disease. Therefore, the treatment goals are essentially palliative and not curative; however, due to its relatively long natural history, many men with metastatic prostate cancer can live for many years and enjoy a reasonably good quality of life, assuming appropriate medical and supportive care are provided.

In the modern era, fewer than 5% of patients in developed nations are diagnosed with *de novo* metastatic prostate cancer. This is attributed to the widespread use of prostate-specific antigen (PSA) screening in these countries. In contrast, a higher proportion of prostate cancer patients in resource-poor nations are diagnosed with advanced disease.

The vast majority of patients with stage 4 prostate cancer present with either nodal or bony metastases. These patients can present with bone pain, or less commonly, discomfort related to tumor bulk, such as urinary obstructive symptoms. Imaging studies, such as bone scintigraphy scans, typically demonstrate uptake over the axial and appendicular skeleton (Fig. 10.1). Rarely, patients may present with lung or liver metastases, easily imaged by standard radiographic techniques such as plain X-rays or computed tomography scans (Figs.10.2 and 10.3). Positron emission tomography (PET) scanning has limited utility in this disease due to the relatively slower growth rate of newly diagnosed prostate cancer (leading to lower FDG-avidity) when compared to other epithelial solid tumors.

Most patients with de novo metastatic prostate cancer have tumors that are androgen-sensitive; that is, these cancer cells are initially dependent on androgen receptor signaling for cell growth and proliferation. This observation has led to the successful exploitation of the endocrine axis as a therapeutic approach (see Chapters 1 and 2).

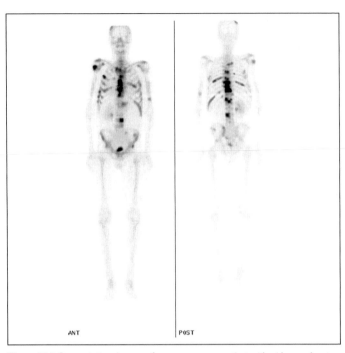

Figure 10.1 Bone scintigraphy scan of a prostate cancer patient with widespread metastasis, showing uptake over the axial and appendicular skeleton

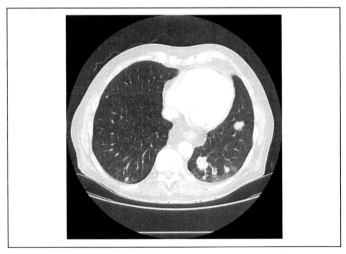

Figure 10.2 Computed tomography scan of a prostate cancer patient with lung metastatic disease

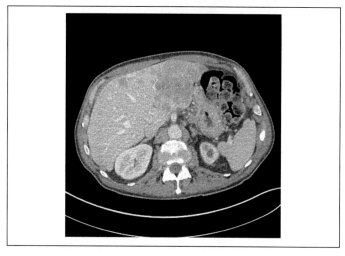

Figure 10.3 Computed tomography scan of a prostate cancer patient with visceral hepatic metastatic disease

Androgen Deprivation Therapy

The principal treatment for metastatic androgen-sensitive prostate cancer is androgen-deprivation (or castration) therapy (ADT). The goal of such therapy is to reduce testicular androgen levels to "castrate levels," traditionally defined as a total serum testosterone level of less than 50 ng/dL, although some advocate for a reduction to even lower levels. Castration therapy results in a clinical benefit—tumor size reduction, PSA reduction, or improvement in symptoms such as bone pain—in over 80% of patients.

Castration can be achieved through either surgical or medical approaches. The primary surgical approach is a bilateral orchiectomy, where the urologist performs a transscrotal procedure to remove both testicles. The alternative approach is "medical castration," which hinges on systemic agents that disrupt hypothalamic-pituitary signaling, a strategy that culminates in the shutdown of luteinizing hormone (LH) outflow from the pituitary gland. Medical castration can be achieved with either an LH releasing-hormone (LHRH) agonist or antagonist. Pituitary LH outflow is governed by the pulsatile secretion of LHRH by the hypothalamus. LHRH agonists such as goserelin or luprolide, often delivered as depot formulations, abrogate native pulsatile signaling, leading to a reduction in LH secretion and subsequently, reduced testosterone output from testicular Leydig cells (Table 10.1).

In contrast, LHRH antagonists such as degarelix compete with natural LHRH for binding to LHRH receptors in the pituitary gland. This reversible binding blocks the release of LH from the pituitary, resulting in medical castration. LHRH agonists and antagonists are delivered as depot formulations, either intramuscularly (e.g., luprolide) or subcutaneously (e.g., goserelin). It must be emphasized that surgical and medical castration strategies are considered

Table 10.1 Select Luteinizing-hormone Releasing-hormone (LHRH) Agonists, LHRH Antagonists, and Androgen Receptor Antagonists

Drug Class	Drug Name	Dose	Route	Schedule	Common Adverse Effects
LHRH Agonists	Goserelin acetate (Zoladex)	10.8 mg	Subcutaneous	Every 12 weeks	Hot flashes, sexual dysfunction, decreased erections, lower urinary tract symptoms, lethargy, pain, edema, upper respiratory infection, rash, and sweating; gynecomastia, pelvic pain, and bone pain have also been reported with higher doses.
	Leuporide acetate (Lupron Depot†)	30 mg	Intramuscular	Every 16 weeks	Hot flashes, general pain, edema, joint disorders, GI disorders, respiratory disorders, urinary disorders, and decreased sexual function.
		22.5 mg	Intramuscular	Every 12 weeks	
		7.5 mg	Intramuscular	Every 4 weeks	
	Triptorelin pamoate (Trelstar)*	22.5 mg	Intramuscular	Every 24 weeks	Hot flashes, skeletal pain, impotence, and headache. Edema, leg pain, erectile dysfunction and testicular atrophy were also commonly reported with higher doses.
		3.75 mg	Intramuscular	Every 4 weeks	
LHRH Antagonists	Degarelix (Firmagon)	240 mg	Subcutaneous	Starting dose of 240 mg given as two subcutaneous injections of 120 mg each followed by monthly maintenance doses of 80 mg given as a single subcutaneous injection	The most common adverse reaction reported with degarelix therapy were injection site reactions (e.g., pain, erythema, swelling or induration), hot flashes, increased weight, fatigue, and increases in serum levels of transaminases and gamma-glutamyltransferase (GGT).
Androgen Receptor Antagonists (Antiandrogens)	Bicalutamide	50 mg	Oral	Once daily	Hot flashes, pain, back pain, asthenia, constipation, pelvic pain, infection, nausea, dyspnea, peripheral edema, diarrhea, hematuria, and nocturia.
	Flutamide	750 mg	Oral	Three times daily	Severe diarrhea was reported more frequently with flutamide treatment compared with LHRH agonist treatment alone.
	Nilutamide	150 mg	Oral	300 mg once a day for 30 days, followed thereafter by 150 mg once a day	Hot flashes, dizziness, constipation, nausea or vomiting, skin rash, loss of appetite, decreased libido, impotence, and vision changes/visual disturbances.

† Leuprolide acetate is also available as a SQ injection (Eligard) in 7.5, 22.5, 30 and 45 mg doses, administered every month, 3 months, 4 months and 6 months, respectively.

* Triptarelin acetate is also available in depot formulation (Trelstar Depot—3.75 mg, administered monthly and as a long-acting injectable suspension (Trelstar LA—11.25 mg, administered every 84 days)

equivalent in terms of survival outcomes, as confirmed by a meta-analysis of randomized trials addressing this issue. The advantages of orchiectomy include its safety, simplicity, and relative cost-effectiveness. However, it is nonreversible and the resulting empty scrotal sac can impose anxiety and other psychological burdens. LHRH agonists or antagonists are easy to administer as depot formulations, possibly reversible, can be delivered on an intermittent basis (see "intermittent therapy" below), but are very expensive.

A surgically castrated patient will not benefit from LHRH agonist or antagonist therapy. However, there are rare instances in which primary medical castration is unable to reduce testicular androgens to castrate levels; in this unusual situation, definitive surgical castration or less commonly, a trial of an alternative LHRH agonist or antagonist can be offered.

It has long been recognized that adrenal androgens, such as androstenedione and dehydroepiandrosterone (DHEA), can also be converted to testosterone (and later to dihydrotestosterone [DHT] by the enzyme 5-α reductase), potentially subverting the reduction of testicular androgen outflow by medical or surgical castration. Thus, agents that block androgen signaling at the androgen receptor (AR) level were developed to address this issue. These so-called *AR antagonists* competitively bind to the AR, hence disrupting AR-mediated growth and proliferation. Androgen receptor antagonists are either steroidal (cyproterone acetate) or nonsteroidal (examples include flutamide, bicalutamide, and nilutamide, among others), and are typically orally bioavailable.

The most common clinical application of AR antagonists is to prevent tumor flare due to transient LH and testosterone surges—lasting for up to 7–14 days—at the initiation of LHRH agonist therapy. This surge is most distressing for patients with bone metastases (where tumor pain increases, or in the case of vertebral metastases, spinal cord compression can occur) or those with an intact prostate gland (where obstructive uropathy is a possibility). To prevent these clinical events, the usual practice for patients at risk for surge-associated complications is to start an AR antagonist 1–2 weeks prior to LHRH agonist therapy, then overlap these agents for an additional 1–2 weeks. Subsequently, single-agent LHRH agonist therapy is pursued (either as continuous or intermittent therapy, as discussed further below). At the time of disease progression (usually manifested by a rise in the serum PSA), some clinicians will initiate AR antagonist therapy simultaneously with LHRH-directed therapy. This strategy will result in disease control only in a modest proportion of patients (refer to Chapter 11: Castration-resistant Prostate Cancer.)

Monotherapy with nonsteroidal AR antagonists has been studied as an alternative to standard castration due to its lower toxicity, particularly with regard to libido preservation. Although a meta-analysis of studies addressing this issue showed that survival is similar between monotherapy nonsteroidal AR antagonists and standard castration, clinical practice has relegated the former only as an alternative to castration for highly selected patients who insist on maintaining libido. In contrast, the data for steroidal antiandrogens as monotherapy is clearer: a randomized trial of the steroidal AR antagonists cyproterone acetate versus goserelin resulted in an inferior time to disease progression for the former compared with the latter.[1]

Single Modality Versus Complete Androgen Blockade

With the availability of AR antagonists, the concept of "complete androgen blockade" emerged, with some clinicians embracing the concept as standard therapy in lieu of single modality (i.e., orchiectomy or LHRH-directed) therapy. This concept is based on combined inhibition of testicular androgen synthesis and the AR, ostensibly to blunt adrenal androgens at the receptor level. Several randomized trials and subsequent meta-analyses of single modality versus complete androgen blockade have since been reported.[2,3,4,5] In sum, these data appear to show that, despite complete androgen blockade resulting in a statistically significant improvement in survival, this improvement was of questionable clinical value or relevance. Considering the additional costs and toxicity of combined therapy over monotherapy—and the very modest (if any) survival benefit—many clinicians presently recommend single-modality therapy for patients with advanced prostate cancer.

Intermittent Versus Continuous Androgen Deprivation

Bilateral orchiectomy—for many decades, the only reliable castration method—is irreversible. When LHRH agonists became available, the duration of therapy mirrored that of surgical castration; that is, they were delivered on a continuous basis until resistance developed or death was imminent. However, as will be discussed later, prolonged castration therapy results in chronic irritative and sometimes unacceptable toxicities. There was also concern that continuous castration may facilitate the development of androgen-independence. Thus, the concept of intermittent androgen deprivation was proposed to help overcome some of the downsides of continuous therapy.[6] Small phase III randomized trials of continuous versus intermittent therapy have already demonstrated that the latter is feasible, associated with improved symptoms and quality of life, may reduce cost, and can result in similar survival outcomes.[7] On a practical basis, these studies show that patients can spend up to 55% of each cycle off therapy when treated with intermittent androgen deprivation. At the time of disease progression, often defined as clinical, radiographic, or biochemical progression (PSA increasing beyond 15–20 ng/dL following an initial nadir), the vast majority of patients have another response following reinstitution of ADT. Standard rules for starting and stopping therapy have not yet been definitively established, but these rules are expected to be defined once the final results of Southwest Oncology Group trial S9346, which randomized patients with advanced prostate cancer to either continuous or intermittent therapy, become available.[8] In the meantime, intermittent therapy is considered by many clinicians to be a reasonable alternative to continuous therapy.

Role of Androgen Deprivation in the High-risk Postprostatectomy Setting

The timing of ADT, as well as the role of systemic chemotherapy in earlier-stage prostate cancer—particularly in the postoperative setting for those deemed at high risk—remains controversial. A small phase III trial (n = 98) from the Eastern Cooperative Oncology Group (ECOG) demonstrated that immediate androgen deprivation improved overall survival in men with node-positive prostate cancer who have undergone radical prostatectomy and pelvic lymphadenectomy, compared with those who received androgen deprivation only at the time of disease progression, with a hazard ratio of 1.84 (95% confidence interval [CI] 1.01–3.35, p = 0.04) in favor of the former. This study established a role for immediate adjuvant ADT in the node-positive, postprostatectomy setting.[9]

The role of immediate postoperative ADT in other high-risk patients is less clear. SWOG 9921 was a prospective, phase III, randomized trial examining the efficacy of adjuvant mitoxantrone chemotherapy in addition to androgen deprivation in a composite group of high-risk patients with prostate cancer. SWOG 9921[10] was closed early due to a higher rate of myeloid leukemia in the chemotherapy arm. However, it must be noted that in that study, "high-risk" patients were defined as having at least one of the following: (1) a pathologic Gleason sum score of 8 or higher; (2) pathologic T3b disease, pT4 disease, or N1 disease; (3) a pathologic Gleason sum score of 7 with a positive surgical margin; or (4) preoperative PSA higher than 15 ng/mL, a biopsy Gleason sum score of 8 or higher, or a PSA of greater than 10 ng/mL with a Gleason sum score of 7 or higher. All patients were required to have an undetectable PSA (≤0.2 ng/mL) before randomization. Final results of this trial remain unavailable.

Toxicities of Androgen Deprivation

Castration therapy is not without toxicity. Symptoms are not unlike those experienced by women undergoing menopause, hence the term *andropause* to describe the symptom complex in men receiving castration therapy. These toxicities include hot flashes, vasomotor instability, irritability, fatigue, loss of libido, sexual dysfunction, gynecomastia, nipple tenderness, and decreased penile size. Among the more concerning side effects are those related to loss of muscle mass, with fatty replacement and weight gain. This has been associated with an increased risk of diabetes and metabolic syndrome. Additionally, castration therapy predisposes men to develop bone loss (osteopenia and/or osteoporosis), which occasionally will result in bone fractures and pain. Patients must be counseled extensively about these toxicities (and their expectations appropriately managed) prior to beginning castration therapy. To prevent or delay some of these toxicities, patients are counseled to remain physically active and to perform weight-bearing exercise, monitor caloric intake to minimize weight gain, and to take calcium (at least 1,000 mg/day of elemental calcium) and vitamin D supplements (at least 400 IU/day). Patients will require baseline and serial monitoring of bone density (DEXA scan); evidence of osteopenia and/or osteoporosis may require initiation of bisphosphonate therapy.

References

1. Seidenfeld J, Damson DJ, Hasselblad V, et al. Single-therapy androgen suppression in men with advanced prostate cancer: A systematic review and meta-analysis. *Ann Intern Med* 2000;132:566–577.

2. Eisenberger MA, Blumenstein BA, Crawford ED, et al. Bilateral orchiectomy with or without flutamide for metastatic prostate cancer. *N Engl J Med* 1998;339:1036–1042.

3. Samson DJ, Seidenfeld J, Schmitt B, et al. Systematic review and meta-analysis of monotherapy compared with combined androgen blockade for patients with advanced prostate carcinoma. *Cancer* 2002;95:361–376.

4. Schmitt B, Wilt TJ, Schellhammer PF. Combined androgen blockade with nonsteroidal antiandrogens for advanced prostate cancer: A systematic review. *Urology* 2001;57:727–732.

5. Prostate Cancer Trialists' Collaborative Group. Maximum androgen blockade in advanced prostate cancer: An overview of the randomised trials. *Lancet* 2000;355:1491–1498.

6. Klotz LH, Herr HW, Morse MJ, et al. Intermittent endocrine therapy for advanced prostate cancer. *Cancer* 1986;58:2546–2550.

7. Abrahamsson PA. Potential benefits of intermittent androgen suppression therapy in the treatment of prostate cancer: a systematic review of the literature. *Eur Urol.* 2010;57(1):49–59.

8. Hussain M, Goldman B, Tangen C, et al. Prostate-specific antigen progression predicts overall survival in patients with metastatic prostate cancer: data from Southwest Oncology Group Trials 9346 (Intergroup Study 0162) and 9916. *J Clin Oncol.* 2009;27(15):2450–6.

9. Messing EM, Manola J, Sarosdy M, et al. Immediate hormonal therapy compared with observation after radical prostatectomy and pelvic lymphadenectomy in men with node-positive prostate cancer. *N Engl J Med* 1999;341:1781–1788.

10. Flaig TW, Tangen CM, Hussain MH, et al. Randomization reveals unexpected acute leukemias in Southwest Oncology Group prostate cancer trial. *J Clin Oncol.* 2008;26(9):1532–6.

Chapter 11

Advanced or Metastatic Prostate Cancer: Castration-resistant Disease

Primo N. Lara, Jr.

Although castration therapy is effective in over 80% of patients with advanced or metastatic prostate cancer, the development of resistance is universal and typically occurs approximately 2 years after castration is initiated. Resistance is thought to occur through either amplification or overexpression of the androgen receptor (AR), mutations in AR, or nonsteroid activation of AR, among others. Castration-resistant prostate cancer (CRPC)—the terminal state of the disease—typically manifests initially as a steady rise in the prostate-specific antigen (PSA) level following a nadir. Radiographic progression will occur approximately 6–12 months after biochemical progression, followed shortly by symptoms including bone pain, weight loss, and increasing fatigue. Occasionally, castration resistance will manifest clinically as symptomatic and radiographic progression rather than simply PSA elevation. Without any therapy at the time of symptomatic or radiographic castration-resistant progression, most patients will succumb to the disease within a year. Thus, these patients are best referred to a medical oncologist for consideration of palliative systemic therapies.

There is no universally accepted definition of CRPC, particularly since some patients with progression while on androgen ablation can still respond to secondary endocrine manipulations. One set of eligibility criteria for clinical trials of CRPC requires that patients have either progressive measurable disease, the presence of at least one new lesion on bone scan, or biochemical progression associated with an increase in PSA, in the presence of castrate levels of testosterone (<50 ng/mL).[1] Progression must occur despite the cessation of treatment with AR antagonists for 4–6 weeks. Biochemical progression is defined as two consecutive increases in PSA from a nadir value, taken at least a week apart each, with a minimum PSA value of 5 ng/mL.

Overview of Systemic Therapies

There is no known curative therapy for CRPC. Hence, the primary goal of any treatment in this disease state is palliative. Systemic therapies attempt to influence the natural history of the disease in order to induce tumor response, prolong such response, and ultimately increase overall survival. Close attention to preservation of quality of life and control of symptoms is essential. Due to the inadequacy of currently available treatments, priority must be given to patient enrollment into investigational clinical trials when available. The following sections address the most commonly offered systemic therapies for CRPC. These include secondary endocrine (hormonal) manipulations, cytotoxic chemotherapy, and investigational therapy. Supportive or ancillary care, including bisphosphonate therapy and radiation/radioisotope therapy, is discussed in a separate chapter.

Endocrine or Hormonal Therapies in the Castration-resistant State

The precise role of continued LHRH agonist or antagonist therapy in CRPC patients who have not undergone prior surgical castration is unclear. Castration-resistant prostate cancer continues to express AR, and thus disease may "flare" with exogenous testosterone administration. A retrospective analysis of patients enrolled in CRPC therapeutic trials found that continued androgen suppression was an important predictor of improved survival. In an analysis of CRPC patients enrolled in phase II chemotherapy trials, those who had prior bilateral orchiectomy appeared to have a median survival time that was 3 months longer than those who had not undergone surgical castration, although the difference did not reach statistical significance.[2] Thus, many clinicians and clinical trialists recommend continuation of androgen deprivation at the time of castration resistance in patients who have not had bilateral orchiectomy. In fact, nearly all clinical trials in CRPC require continuation of LHRH agonist or antagonist therapy for those nonorchiectomized patients while on study. Often, castration therapy is eventually discontinued at the time of hospice enrollment.

In medically or surgically castrated patients who have not had prior exposure to an antiandrogen, or who have had only brief prior therapy with an antiandrogen to prevent a surge, the addition of an antiandrogen at the time of castration resistance may benefit some patients. In general, approximately 13%–30% of patients can potentially respond to the addition of antiandrogen therapy in this setting. This "response" is usually in the form of a PSA decline. These data favor the use of agents such as bicalutamide when antiandrogen therapy is contemplated.

On the other hand, there are patients who are already on complete androgen blockade who have biochemical or clinical evidence of castration resistance. In this patient cohort, discontinuation of the antiandrogen may be therapeutic. It is thought that aberrant activation of the AR by the antiandrogen results in renewed signaling through AR-responsive pathways. Up to 33% of patients have been reported to respond to withdrawal of flutamide or other antiandrogens. This response occurs within 8 weeks and has been reported to last from 3 to 14 months. This so-called *antiandrogen withdrawal response* is widely recognized; in fact, clinical trials in CRPC require that all patients must have any antiandrogens discontinued and any postwithdrawal response must be assessed prior to study entry. Unfortunately, there is no evidence that antiandrogen withdrawal prolongs overall patient survival.

Several other second-line endocrine manipulation agents have also been reported in CRPC, including diethylstilbestrol, tamoxifen, megestrol, aminoglutethimide, and corticosteroids. A wide range of PSA responses has been reported with these agents, but the response duration is generally less than 6 months.[3]

Ketoconazole is an orally bioavailable antifungal agent that also decreases adrenal steroid synthesis through inhibition of LY19 and CYP17. This mechanism of action results in a reduction in the production of adrenal androgen species, such as androstenedione and DHEA, which can be converted to testosterone and thence activate the AR. The usual ketoconazole dose that results in sufficient adrenal suppression is much higher (400 mg orally three times daily) than that used for its antifungal activity. Because of its adrenal suppressive properties, ketoconazole is usually administered with hydrocortisone at 30 mg orally in the morning and 10 mg orally in the late afternoon. Prostate-specific antigen (PSA) response rates of 50% or higher have been reported in studies of ketoconazole plus hydrocortisone. A cooperative group randomized trial of antiandrogen withdrawal alone versus antiandrogen withdrawal plus high-dose ketoconazole with hydrocortisone (with crossover to ketoconazole at progression in the control arm) demonstrated a significantly higher PSA response rate in the ketoconazole arm (27% versus 13%) but also with a higher proportion of grade 3 or 4 toxicities with ketoconazole. There was no survival difference, likely to due the crossover design.[4]

Abiraterone acetate is an adrenal androgen inhibitor that irreversibly inhibits 17-α hydroxylase and C17,20-lyase and hence decreases adrenal androgen production. It has emerged as a highly active agent in both chemotherapy-naïve as well as chemotherapy pretreated CRPC patients. Phase III placebo-controlled trials testing abiraterone in CRPC have already been completed. In one of these studies (COU-AA-301), 1,195 patients with metastatic CRPC whose disease had progressed following treatment with one or two chemotherapy regimens, at least one of which contained docetaxel, were randomized to either abiraterone/prednisone versus placebo/prednisone. At interim analysis this trial was reported to have a statistically significant improvement in overall survival – the primary endpoint - in favor of the abiraterone arm.

MDV3100 is a novel nonsteroidal antiandrogen that binds to AR with higher affinity than bicalutamide. It also reduces nuclear translocation of the AR complex, thus preventing AR elements in DNA from being activated. In early-phase trials of MDV3100, a substantial proportion of CRPC patients (whether chemotherapy-naive or -pretreated) experienced biochemical (PSA) or radiographic response. MDV3100 is under evaluation in the CRPC setting.

Immunotherapy

Among the more interesting new agents against CRPC is sipuleucel-T (Provenge), an immunologic product that utilizes antigen-presenting cells (specifically dendritic cells) loaded with antigen ex vivo to stimulate a T-cell immune response.[5] Sipuleucel-T is manufactured by fusing human prostatic acid phosphatase (PAP) to a granulocyte-macrophage colony-stimulating factor (GM-CSF) cassette, which is thought to facilitate internalization and presentation of the PAP antigen. Dendritic cells are obtained from the patients through leukocytapheresis and then sent to the vaccine manufacturer for processing. A randomized phase III study of sipuleucel-T in men with metastatic CRPC showed that sipuleucel-T prolonged median survival by 4.1 months and improved 3-year survival by 38% as compared to placebo, with a reduction in the risk of death by 22.5% ($p = 0.032$). Common adverse reactions reported in clinical trials were chills, fatigue, fever, back pain, nausea, joint ache, and headache. These data led to the U.S. Food and Drug Administration (FDA) approval of sipuleucel-T for CRPC therapy.

Chemotherapy

Cytotoxic chemotherapy plays a substantial role in the palliative management of advanced CRPC. The first chemotherapeutic agent to receive FDA approval in this indication was the anthracenedione mitoxantrone (Novantrone). A phase III trial of mitoxantrone plus prednisone versus prednisone alone, designed with a unique endpoint of palliative response, showed that significantly more patients treated with mitoxantrone experienced palliation (29% versus 12%, $p = 0.01$), and that the duration of palliation was also significantly longer (43 versus 18 weeks, $p <0.0001$).[6] A second trial (Cancer and Leukemia Group B [CALGB] study 9182), compared mitoxantrone plus hydrocortisone to hydrocortisone alone. Patients treated with mitoxantrone had delayed time to disease progression and a trend toward improved quality of life.[7] The recommended dose of mitoxantrone in CRPC is 12 to 14 mg/m^2 given as a short intravenous infusion every 21 days. Common side effects reported include nausea, alopecia, neutropenia, diarrhea, fatigue, and constipation, among others.

The taxane docetaxel (Taxotere) has an established role in the standard frontline management of previously untreated CRPC patients. Southwest Oncology Group (SWOG) trial S9916[8] showed that the combination of docetaxel/prednisone plus estramustine significantly improves survival over mitoxantrone plus prednisone. TAX 327, a randomized trial of two different schedules (weekly or every 3 week) of docetaxel plus prednisone compared to mitoxantrone/prednisone demonstrated improved survival in favor of the every-3-week docetaxel dose schedule (docetaxel 75 mg/m^2 every 3 weeks plus 5 mg oral prednisone twice daily).[9] Subsequent clinical trials that have attempted to improve on the efficacy of docetaxel in this setting by adding an investigational agent (in combination with docetaxel versus docetaxel alone) have thus far failed. Notably, these agents include the angiogenesis inhibitor bevacizumab and the vitamin

D-based agent DN-101 (high-dose calcitriol). In prostate cancer, docetaxel is indicated in combination with prednisone and the recommended dose is is 75 mg/m^2 every 3 weeks as a 1 hour intravenous infusion. Prednisone 5 mg orally BID is administered continuously. Common adverse effects reported included bone marrow suppression, sensory neuropathy, alopecia, nail changes, tearing, fluid retetion, and fatigue, among others.

In CRPC patients who have failed prior chemotherapy, a phase III trial of the novel taxane cabazitaxel (Jevtana) plus prednisone versus mitoxantrone plus prednisone demonstrated statistically improved overall survival in favor of cabazitaxel-based therapy.[10] This trial demonstrated the ability of cabazitaxel to potentially overcome taxane-resistance in the second-line setting. On the strength of these data, cabazitaxel was approved by the FDA for the treatment (in combination with prednisone) of CRPC patients in the post-docetaxel setting. The recommended dose is 25 mg/m^2 administered every three weeks as a one-hour intravenous infusion in combination with oral prednisone 10 mg administered daily throughout cabazitaxel treatment. Common side effects include bone marrow suppression (neutropenia, anemia, leukopenia, and thrombocytopenia), diarrhea, fatigue/asthenia, peripheral neuropathy, arthralgia, and alopecia, among others.

In the context of suboptimal outcomes following systemic therapy, patients with CRPC are encouraged to consider investigational therapies (within organized clinical trials) as a reasonable therapeutic option.

References

1. G.J. Bubley, M. Carducci, W. Dahut, N. Dawson, D. Daliani, M. Eisenberger et al., Eligibility and response guidelines for phase II clinical trials in androgen-independent prostate cancer: recommendations from the Prostate-Specific Antigen Working Group. *J. Clin. Oncol.* 17 11 (1999), pp. 3461–3467. View Record in Scopus | Cited By in Scopus (515).

2. Hussain M, Wolf M, Marshall E, et al. Effects of continued androgen-deprivation therapy and other prognostic factors on response and survival in phase II chemotherapy trials for hormone-refractory prostate cancer: A Southwest Oncology Group report. *J Clin Oncol* 1994;12(9);1868–1875.

3. Martel CL, Gumerlock PH, Meyers FJ, Lara PN Jr. Current strategies in the management of hormone refractory prostate cancer. *Cancer Treat Rev* 2003;29:171–187.

4. Small EJ, Halabi S, Dawson NA, et al. Antiandrogen withdrawal alone or in combination with ketoconazole in androgen-independent prostate cancer patients: A phase III trial (CALGB 9583). *J Clin Oncol* 2004;22(6):1025–1033.

5. Kantoff, P., Higano CS, Berger ER, et al. Updated survival results of the IMPACT trial of sipuleucel-T for metastatic castration resistant prostate cancer. *2010 Genitourinary Cancers Symposium Proceedings* 2010;[Abstract] 8:65.

6. Tannock IF, Osoba D, Stockler MR, et al. Chemotherapy with mitoxantrone plus prednisone or prednisone alone for symptomatic hormone-resistant prostate cancer: A Canadian randomized trial with palliative end points. *J Clin Oncol* 1996;14:1756–1764.

7. Kantoff PW, Halabi S, Conaway M, et al. Hydrocortisone with or without mitoxantrone in men with hormone-refractory prostate cancer: Results of the Cancer and Leukemia Group B 9182 study. *J Clin Oncol* 1999;17:2506–2513.

8. Petrylak DP, Tangen CM, Hussain MH, et al. Docetaxel and estramustine compared with mitoxantrone and prednisone for advanced refractory prostate cancer. *N Engl J Med* 2004;351(15):1513–1520.

9. Tannock IF, de Wit R, Berry WR, et al. Docetaxel plus prednisone or mitoxantrone plus prednisone for advanced prostate cancer. *N Engl J Med* 2004; 351(15):1502–1512.

10. J. S. De Bono, S. Oudard, M. Ozguroglu, et al. Cabazitaxel or mitoxantrone with prednisone in patients with metastatic castration-resistant prostate cancer (mCRPC) previously treated with docetaxel: Final results of a multinational phase III trial (TROPIC). *J Clin Oncol* 2010;28:15s: [Abstract]4508.

Chapter 12

Supportive Therapies for Prostate Cancer

Primo N. Lara, Jr.

Appropriate supportive care is essential for prostate cancer patients, particularly with regard to the management of side effects from local or systemic therapy. In patients with advanced refractory prostate cancer for whom reasonable tumor-directed care has been exhausted, aggressive palliative care—ideally delivered in the context of a licensed hospice program—should always be a principal consideration. This chapter addresses the various ancillary or supportive therapies available to the prostate cancer patient, with emphasis on clinically validated strategies.

Bone Health

Bone is remodeled throughout life and is distinguished by a balance between renewed formation by osteoblasts and mineral resorption initiated by osteoclasts. The coupling of these two processes is important in the maintenance of normal bone turnover.

It is already well known that androgen deprivation therapy (ADT), either by surgical or medical means, induces or accelerates osteoporosis and osteopenia. Other factors contribute to bone loss in prostate cancer patients, including diet, lifestyle, or direct involvement of the skeleton with metastatic prostate cancer deposits.

One hypothesis for the increase in resorption associated with bone metastases is that the cancer cells secrete factors (e.g., parathyroid hormone-related peptide [PTH-rp]) that directly stimulate osteoclastic bone resorption.[1] In response, the skeleton releases factors such as tumor growth factor-β, which then stimulate the tumor cells to produce bone resorptive factors such as PTH-rp. This ultimately results in a vicious cycle of bone resorption.[2] This increased bone turnover (from whatever cause) results in diminished bone integrity, ultimately causing the devastating clinical features of bone pain, fractures, and hypercalcemia, otherwise called *skeletal-related events* (SREs). It is estimated that approximately 49% of patients with prostate cancer and bone metastases will experience an SRE without treatment and that, in these men, median time to first SRE is less than 11 months.[3]

Men with prostate cancer initiating androgen deprivation must be apprised of the increased risk of SREs during the course of such therapy. Similar to postmenopausal women, monitoring of bone density with dual-energy X-ray absorptiometry (DEXA) scans in these men is reasonable, as is supplementation with elemental calcium of at least 1,000 mg/day orally and vitamin D of at least 400 IU/day orally. Patients are also encouraged to continue weight-bearing exercise.

As osteopenia and osteoporosis become more prevalent with the use of early androgen blockade, the use of bisphosphonates as adjunctive therapy has increased. Bisphosphonates are typically used to treat hypercalcemia, but they also have potent antiresorptive and bone stabilizing activity, making them ideal agents to manage bone health in men with prostate cancer. Oral agents, such as alendronate (Fosamax), can reduce the rate of bone mineral loss in men with osteoporosis, whereas the intravenous agent pamidronate disodium (Aredia) has been shown to reduce the rate of bone mineral loss in men without bone metastases who are treated with androgen ablation. In a phase III placebo-controlled randomized clinical trial in castration-resistant prostate cancer patients, zoledronic acid (Zometa) delivered at 4 mg intravenously once a month was shown to significantly reduce the rate of SREs. Specifically, zoledronic acid extended median time to first SRE by more than 5 months and reduced the risk of SREs by 36% as compared to placebo. However, the use of bisphosphonates is also associated with certain unique adverse events, including esophagitis (for oral agents), renal dysfunction, and osteonecrosis of the jaw (ONJ).

The effect of the monoclonal antibody denosumab, which targets the receptor activator of nuclear factor-κB ligand, on bone mineral density and fractures in men receiving ADT for nonmetastatic prostate cancer has also been investigated.[4] In a double-blind, multicenter placebo-controlled study, bone mineral density of the lumbar spine was found to be increased by 5.6% in the denosumab group, as compared with a loss of 1.0% in the placebo group (p <0.001). Denosumab therapy was also associated with a decreased incidence of new vertebral fractures at 36 months.

A randomized phase III trial of monthly denosumab versus zoledronic acid in over 1,900 men with castration-resistant prostate cancer and at least one bone metastasis has also been conducted.[5] In this trial, SREs were defined as pathologic fracture, radiation, or surgery to bone, or spinal cord compression. Denosumab was given at a dose of 120 mg subcutaneously once every 4 weeks. In that trial, denosumab significantly delayed the time to first on-study SRE as compared with zoledronic acid, with a hazard ratio of 0.82 (p = 0.008). Median time to first on-study SRE was 20.7 months in the denosumab arm and 17.1 in the zoledronic acid arm. Although toxicities were fairly comparable, ONJ was higher with denosumab as compared to zoledronic acid (2.3% vs. 1.3%). Denosumab (Xgeva) was recently approved for the prevention of skeletal-related events from solid tumors. The recommended dosage is 120 mg every 4 weeks as a subcutaneous injection in the upper arm, upper thigh, or abdomen (to be co-administered with calcium and vitamin D as necessary to treat or prevent hypocalcemia). The most common adverse reactions (incidence greater than or equal to 25%) were fatigue/asthenia, hypophosphatemia, and nausea.

Bone Pain: Narcotic, Radioisotope, and Palliative Radiation Therapy

Since bone metastases are a very common clinical event in prostate cancer, it is not surprising that bone pain due to metastatic disease is also a typical clinical issue for these patients. Oral analgesic therapy is often effective in treating pain due to bone metastases. Non-narcotic options such nonsteroidal anti-inflammatory drugs (e.g., ibuprofen or naproxen sodium) appear to have better (albeit anecdotal) efficacy for bone pain over acetaminophen. Narcotics (opioid-based, such as morphine or methadone) are required to treat moderate to severe bone pain and are often prescribed for both long-acting maintenance (round-the-clock) and/or rescue (as-needed) indications.

In patients with advanced prostate cancer, external beam radiation is sometimes an option to treat symptoms related to local disease progression, such as hematuria, pelvic pain, or urinary obstruction. It can also prevent pathologic fractures due to bone metastases if administered before the cortex is eroded by greater than 50%, and may completely eliminate bone pain in up to 75% of patients. Unfortunately, for patients with extensive bone disease or many previously irradiated sites, complete pain relief is less likely.

The β-emitting radioisotopes, such as ^{32}Phosphorus and ^{89}Strontium, and the mixed β- and γ-emitter ^{153}Samarium have long been employed to treat painful bone metastases.[6,7] ^{32}Phosphorus therapy results in pain relief in 70%–90% of patients within 2 weeks, but is associated with substantial myelosuppression. ^{89}Strontium and ^{153}Samarium are both predominantly taken up by regions of increased osteoblastic activity, notably in sites of metastatic disease. It has been reported that up to 80% will achieve at least partial pain relief with these radioisotopes, with 10% becoming pain-free. The duration of pain response is fairly modest, lasting approximately 3–6 months. Retreatment with another dose of radioisotopes is an option, but these subsequent therapies are limited by suboptimal bone marrow tolerance. In a randomized trial comparing ^{89}Strontium with local or hemibody external beam radiation, incidence and duration of pain relief was found to be similar. However, ^{89}Strontium-treated patients were less likely to report new sites of pain, and need for further external beam radiation was less likely after ^{89}Strontium therapy than after local radiation.

Sexual Dysfunction

The most common form of sexual dysfunction in the prostate cancer patient is erectile dysfunction (ED), defined as the inability to develop or sustain an erection satisfactory for sexual intercourse. Most often, ED is not directly due to prostate cancer but rather as a consequence of toxicity of treatment for prostate cancer. These treatments include surgery (robotic or radical prostatectomy), radiation therapy, cryotherapy, and ADT, among others. Not all patients will experience permanent ED; the rate and severity is influenced in part by patient age and comorbidities, quality of preoperative erections, type of surgery, radiation dosimetry and plan, disease stage, and experience of the surgeon.

Erectile dysfunction will universally occur after a prostatectomy, with gradual recovery thereafter. A nerve-sparing prostatectomy technique usually results in recovery from ED within the first year following the procedure. In those who did not undergo a nerve-sparing procedure, erectile function is unlikely to return. In patients who undergo primary radiation therapy, ED onset is typically gradual, beginning approximately 6 months following the treatment. However, radiation-associated ED is less common with more modern treatments, such as radioactive seed implants (brachytherapy), intensity-modulated radio-therapy (IMRT), and 3D conformal radiotherapy. In patients receiving ADT, loss of libido is the most common culprit for ED. Treatment options for ED include orally bioavailable phosphodiesterase-PDE5 inhibitors, such as sildena-fil or tadalafil; vasodilator therapy with the prostaglandin (PGE-1) alprostadil delivered either by intracavernous injection or urethral suppository; vacuum constriction devices; and surgically implanted penile prosthetic implants. A con-sultation with an ED specialist—usually a subspecialized urologic surgeon—is highly recommended for these patients.

Incontinence

Urinary incontinence is a common adverse event of therapy for localized pros-tate cancer and is associated with a suboptimal quality of life. Postprostatectomy incontinence when loosely defined as *any* form of leakage, has been reported in up to 70% of cases. Incontinence occurring after primary radiation therapy is less common but is not a rare event. Supportive management depends on incontinence type (either stress, overflow, or urge), patient comorbidities, and patient desires. A comprehensive discussion of the therapeutic modalities for incontinence is beyond the scope of this book. Treatment options include Kegel exercises, biofeedback, anticholinergics, collagen injections, indwelling urinary catheters, and surgically implanted artificial sphincters, among others.

References

1. Guise TA. Parathyroid hormone-related protein and bone metastases. *Cancer* 1997;80(8 Suppl):1572–1580.

2. Mundy GR. Mechanisms of bone metastasis. *Cancer* 1997;80(8 Suppl):1546–1556.

3. Saad F, Gleason DM, Murray R, et al. Long-term efficacy of zoledronic acid for the prevention of skeletal complications in patients with metastatic hormone-refractory prostate cancer. *J Natl Cancer Inst* 2004;96:879–882.

4. Smith MR Egerdie B, Toriz NH, et al. Denosumab in men receiving androgen-deprivation therapy for prostate cancer. *N Engl J Med* 2009; (8):745–755.

5. Fizazi K, Carducci MA, Smith MR, et al. A randomized phase III trial of denosumab versus zoledronic acid in patients with bone metastases from castration resistant prostate cancer. *J Clin Oncol* 2010;28(18s):951s, LBA4507.

6. Pandit-Taskar, N, Batraki M, Divgi CR. Radiopharmaceutical therapy for palliation of bone pain from osseous metastases. *J Nucl Med* 2004;45(8):1358–1365.

7. Hamdy NA, Papapoulos SE. The palliative management of skeletal metastases in prostate cancer: use of bone-seeking radionuclides and bisphosphonates. (2001). *Semin Nucl Med* 2001;31(1):62–68.

Index